AF385715

Frontiers in European Radiology

8

Editors-in-Chief

A. L. Baert · F. H. W. Heuck

Editorial Board

L. Dalla-Palma · P. Dawson · L. Diankov · G. du Boulay
R. Günther · G. Kalifa · J. Lammer · M. Laval-Jeantet
R. Passariello · C. Pedrosa · H. Pokieser · M. Reiser
J. Remy · W. Semmler · U. Speck
C. Standertskjöld-Nordenstam · H. Thomsen
A. Valavanis · D. Vanel · P. F. G. M. van Waes · P. Vock

Founding Editors

Albert L. Baert · Erik Boijsen
Walter A. Fuchs · Friedrich H. W. Heuck

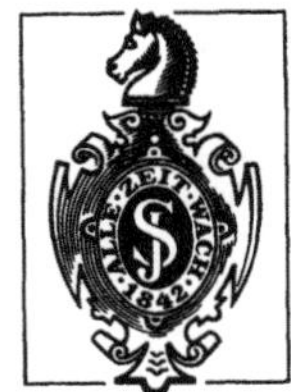

Springer-Verlag

Berlin Heidelberg New York
London Paris Tokyo
Hong Kong Barcelona
Budapest

Professor Dr. A.L. Baert
Katholieke Universiteit Leuven,
Universitaire Ziekenhuizen Gasthuisberg,
Dienst Radiologie, B-3000 Leuven

Professor Dr. F.H.W. Heuck
Director emeritus, Radiologisches Institut,
Katharinenhospital Stuttgart
Private address:
Hermann-Kurz-Straße 5, D-7000 Stuttgart 1

Founding Editors:
Albert L. Baert · Erik Boijsen ·
Walter A. Fuchs · Friedrich H.W. Heuck

With 49 Figures and 9 Tables

ISBN-13:978-3-642-76101-0   e-ISBN-13:978-3-642-76099-0
DOI: 10.1007/978-3-642-76099-0

Typesetting: Thomson Press (India) Ltd, New Delhi

21/3020-543210 - Printed on acid-free paper

Contents

Progress in Biomagnetic Imaging of Heart Arrhythmias

W. Moshage[1], S. Achenbach[1], A. Weikl[1], K. Göhl[1], K. Abraham-Fuchs[2], S. Schneider[2] and K. Bachmann[1]

1 Introduction

In industrial nations today, there are, per million inhabitants, about 2000–3000 deaths caused by cardiac problems every year [12]. Since half of these cases result from different types of arrhythmias, it is clear that a simple, fast, and noninvasive method is needed to thoroughly investigate these diseases in the early stages of development.

One disorder which is inadequately supported from a diagnostic and therapeutic standpoint is the Wolf–Parkinson–White syndrome (WPW syndrom). The incidence of this disease is reported to be between 0.1% and 0.3%, which means that there are 1000–3000 patients per million inhabitants. The mortality of this group is about 2.25 times higher than that of the average population [13]. Patients who are at especially high risk are those with spontaneous orthodromic or antidromic tachycardia. When drug treatment is unsuccessful, it is necessary to precisely

---

[1] *Medical Clinic II (Cardiology) and Policlinic, University Erlangen-Nuremberg, FRG*
[2] Siemens AG, Medical Eng. Group, Erlangen, FRG

Frontiers in European Radiology, Vol. 8
Eds. Baert/Heuck
© Springer-Verlag, Berlin Heidelberg 1991

localize the accessory pathways in order that interventional therapy such as catheter ablation or surgical interruption of the arrhythmogenic bundle can be applied.

The accurate localization of electrical activity within the heart is particularly important in patients with coronary disease. The risk of sudden cardiac death in patients recovering from myocardial infarction increases with the occurrence of complex arrhythmias [17], the incidence ranging from 0.4‰ per year in patients under 45 years old up to 7.2‰ per year in patients over 75 years old [12]. The reason for sudden cardiac death (up to 90%) has been documented as ventricular fibrillation which, in most cases, is preceded by ventricular tachycardia [16].

Historically, the localization of electrical activity in the heart was only possible using complex invasive catheter techniques. Up to five catheters carrying several electrodes had to be placed in the right and/or left heart, the entire procedure usually taking several hours. For the two groups of patients mentioned, a noninvasive and fast method of investigation which imposes minimal strain on the patient seems highly desirable.

2 Principles of Biomagnetic Localization

Activity of biological cells such as nerves and muscle fibers is electric in origin. In a physical context, excited cells can be considered as galvanic elements situated in a conductive medium—the body; sometimes bundles of cells are active at the same time. These cells can be modeled as an equivalent current dipole, consisting of a current source and sink separated by a short distance.

A current dipole (i.e., a small battery) sends volume current into the conductive surrounding. When these currents reach the surface of the body, electric potentials can be measured with electrodes. In medical diagnosis measurements in the head are shown on an electroencephalogram (EEG) and those in the heart are shown on an electrocardiogram (ECG). EEGs and ECGs provide information on the time course of the current sources in the body. However, localization is not possible using these signals due to the strong influence of local tissue conductivity, which can vary considerably.

The strength of these electric fields generally depends on the strength of the source and on the position of the electrodes with respect to the source. Since the conductivity of different tissues normally is not known, localization of a current dipole in the body is only possible with electrodes if they are brought very close to the site of the electric activity. To determine the origin of electric activity in the human heart one therefore has to work with catheters—an invasive procedure.

It is well known that every electric current is surrounded by a magnetic field which is, in essence, unaffected by the electromagnetic properties of the tissue. Research into the localization of current dipoles using magnetic field measurements was performed as early as 1963 [2]. The magnetic field, generated by a current dipole in the human body and measured outside of the body, has two fields of activity: one originates from the current dipole itself and the other originates from the volume currents. While the influence of the first field of activity can easily be calculated from the Biot–Savart law, the second depends on the paths of the currents in the body.

The influence of the volume currents can be quantitatively taken into account if the geometry of the body is known. Modeling using simple structures permits analytical treatment. The simplest models are an infinite half-space for the chest and a sphere for the head [4]. It turns out that volume currents contribute to the magnetic field much less than the current dipole itself. For this reason biomagnetic localization yields satisfactory results even though shape and conductivity of the human body is only crudely taken into account.

In order to localize the current dipole it is necessary to know the magnetic field distribution. Generally, one measures a north pole where the magnetic field lines leave the human body, and a south pole where they enter again (Figs. 5, 8). The current dipole lies in the center between these two poles. The depth is determined by the distance between the two poles; the further the two poles are apart, the deeper the dipole is situated.

A specific determination of the three-dimensional position of the dipole from the measured field distribution is only possible using an iterative process. Based on a first approximation of the dipole position, the field distribution is calculated; for the heart embedded in the thorax the simple model of the infinite half-space is used. The distribution calculated and measured field are then compared and the locus of the dipole altered until minimum deviation in measurements is reached; the point of minimum deviation is then considered as the location of the electric source.

3 The Multichannel Biomagnetic Measurement System

Biomagnetic fields are six to eight orders of magnitude smaller than the earth's magnetic field as shown in Table 1. Their measurement requires considerable efforts to suppress interference from external fields in order to reach the necessary sensitivity.

For the last decade biomagnetic investigations have been carried out utilizing systems with only a few channels [5, 7, 14, 15] and since knowledge of a sufficiently large field map is required for localization of biomagnetic sources, measurements had to be made sequentially, or point by point. This meant that measurement times

Table 1. Magnitudes of biomagnetic and noise fields

Magnetic activity	Field strength	
Evoked cortical activity	50	fT
MEG spontaneous activity (α, δ)	1	pT
MCG (R wave)	50	pT
Magnetized lung contaminants	1	nT
Geomagnetic activity	0.1	nT
Urban noise	10–100	nT
Earth field	50	μT

MEG, Magnetoencephalogram; MCG, magnetocardiogram

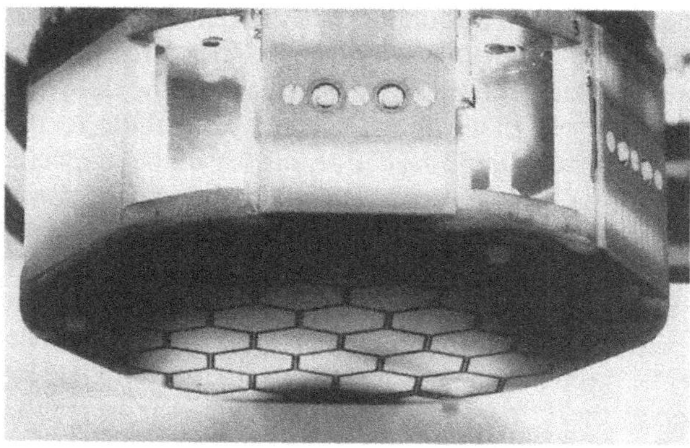

Fig. 1. Array of 37 axial first-order gradiometers

could last several hours or more. Furthermore, field distributions of spontaneous events could not be measured at all.

The Krenikon [11] was the first large-scale biomagnetic multichannel system used routinely for patient studies. To prevent interference from external electromagnetic fields, measurements are taken in a shielded room constructed of conductive and soft magnetic material. The measurement system consists of 37 superconducting detection coils and 37 compensation coils arranged on flat disks 19 cm in diameter and 7 cm apart (Fig. 1). These coils are linked to silicon chips with integrated superconducting quantum interference devices (SQUIDs). This arrangement is placed in a cryostat (insulating container) filled with liquid helium. The cryostat can be adjusted vertically and titled in two directions, which together with adjustment of the patient couch allows easy and precise patient positioning within the measurement field.

With biomagnetic multichannel systems, a magnetic field distribution can be acquired with an acquisition rate up to 6000 Hz (depending on the application). From the resulting field maps, electric current dipoles can be successively localized in three dimensions for each instant in time. These positions can be projected onto three orthogonal planes, where they give an image of the propagation of the current dipole (Fig. 4). Dipole locations and propagation can also be fused with diagnostic images acquired by magnetic resonance imaging (MRI) or computed tomography (CT). The combination of biomagnetism and multichannel systems thus opens new avenues in the analysis of biological function, with a time resolution unrivaled by any other method. We will refer to this procedure as biomagnetic imaging.

4 Performing a Biomagnetic Investigation

Routine preparation for an actual patient measurement takes only a few minutes. The patient removes all magnetic materials such as belt, jewelry, watch, etc. before an investigation can be performed. Nonmagnetic ECG electrodes and a respiration belt are then applied. The patient is placed on the examination table and the ECG electrodes and respiration belt are then connected to the electronics.

For a biomagnetic investigation one needs a fixed reference system, which is provided by a plastic support with four small wire coils taped to the patient's chest. The exact position of the coils are marked with a pen on the chest. The dewar is brought to a distance of a few centimeters above the coils and constant current is run through one coil after another; the respective magnetic fields are recorded. At this point the localization coils and holder are removed and the sensor (dewar) is placed in position above the patient's chest — as close as respiratory movement will allow (Fig. 2). This repositioning of the dewar is measured and registered.

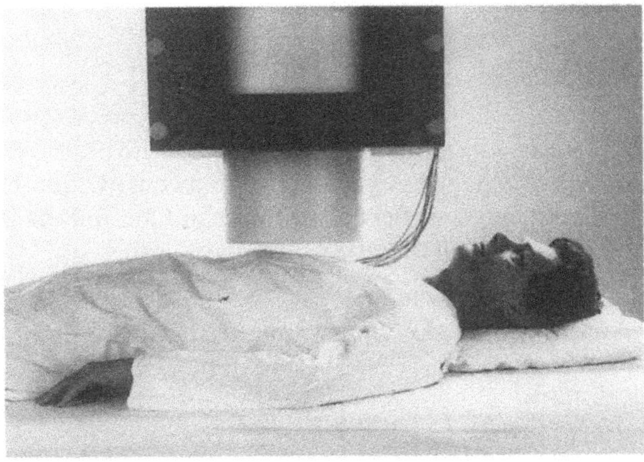

Fig. 2. Arrangement for MCG measurement with simultaneous ECG recording

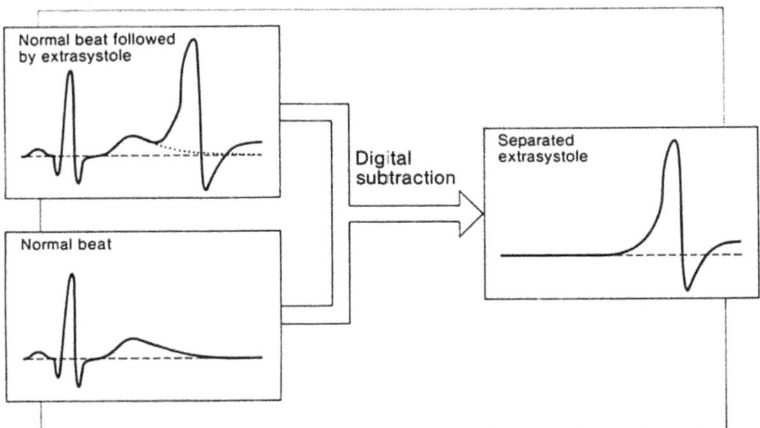

Fig. 3. Schematic representation of digital subtraction performed in the case of an extrasystole emerging from the repolarization of a normal beat. Averaged normal beats are subtracted from the combination of a normal beat followed by an extrasystole to obtain the isolated extrasystole. This procedure is carried out in each channel separately

The actual data acquisition is then begun due to the fact that the sensor array is 19 cm in diameter, no serial measurement or repositioning of the patient is necessary. In addition to the signals from the magnetic channels, i.e., MCG, ECG and respiration is also recorded. This allows the correlation of electrical and magnetic signals and the identification of artifacts due to respiration. Typical measurement times are 4–10 min. After data acquisition is complete, the dewar is brought back to the first measurement position and the plastic support is applied again in order to check whether the patient has moved.

Normally, an ECG-triggered multislice MR investigation follows. In order to establish a common reference system for the biomagnetic and MR images, the aforementioned plastic support is also used in MRI, but the wire coils are now replaced by tiny tubes filled with contrast agent. These tubes can be easily identified in the MR images.

5 Evaluation of Data

The end result of data evaluation in biomagnetic imaging is the reconstruction of bioelectric activity from the measured magnetic field distribution in time and space (Fig. 4). This procedure consists of several signal-processing steps:

— Baseline correction in each measurement channel
— Optional averaging of several heart cycles to improve the signal-to-noise ratio (SNR)
— Definition of a physiological model
— Source reconstruction
— Semi-automated validation of the reconstruction result
— Visualization of the reconstructed three dimensional localization of the bioelectric activity by fusion with other imaging methods

Biomagnetic image reconstruction is critically dependent on signal fidelity. Signal distortions, such as dc offset and low frequency (i.e., below 0.1 Hz) noise, have to be removed without imposing new distortions. Dc offset and low frequency noise stems mainly from electronic noise in high-gain amplifiers, thermal magnetic noise in surrounding materials, respiratory movement of the torso, and mechanical vibrations. In some cases the baseline of a signal of interest is also influenced by a preceding physiological activity. Special correction algorithms have been developed for these cases and depending on the type of pathology under study, different baseline correction techniques are applied.

1. The simplest correction algorithm makes use of the fact that the heart is electrically inactive during the T–P interval of the heart cycle. A time window preceding the P wave is defined and the mean of the signal during this interval is subtracted from the total signal for each channel individually.
2. Sometimes the baseline of intermittent pathological activity is overlapped by the activity of a preceding normal heartbeat, as is the case when an extrasystole emerges from the end of the T wave of the preceding heartbeat. In this case, the

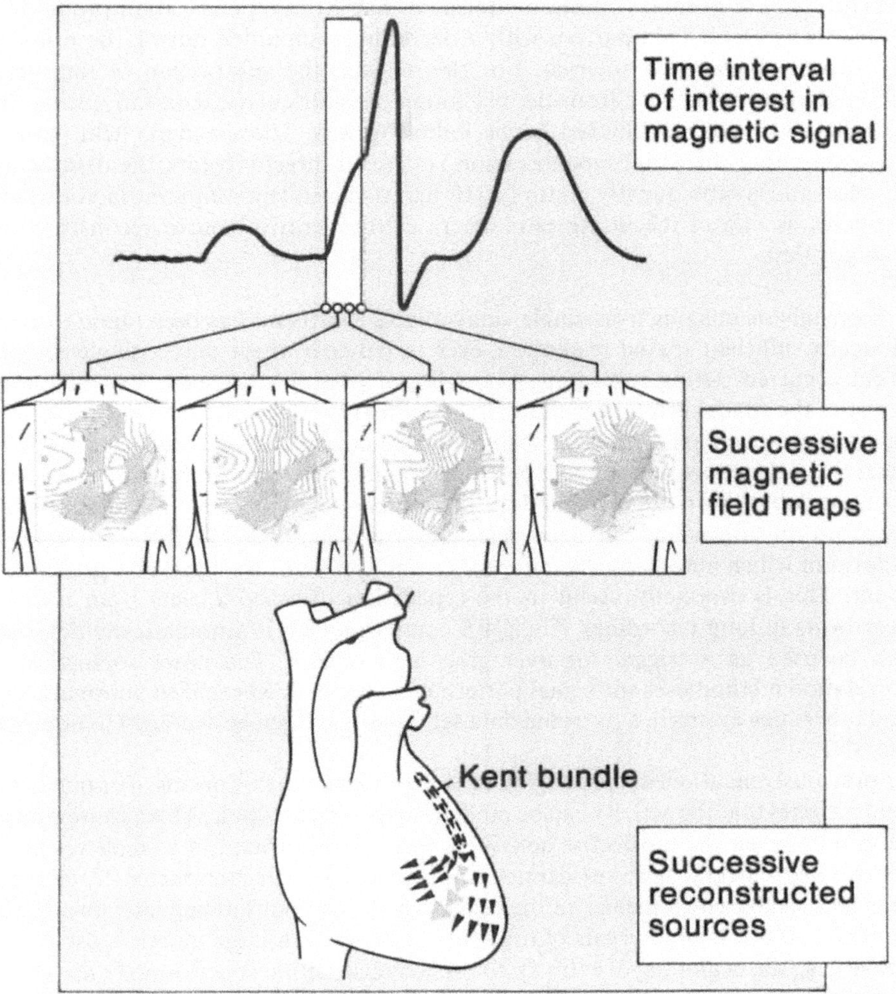

Fig. 4. Schematic representation of source reconstruction from successive field maps, Source localization during time window of interest (*shaded in white*) yields successive source locations (*yellow arrows*), representing the center of the spreading excitation wavefront. (Example of Kent's bundle localization)

average of a few (or even a single) normal heartbeats provides a template which represents the baseline distortion during an extrasystole. The template is then subtracted from the normal heartbeat preceding the extrasystole after fine alignment via cross-correlation (Fig. 3).

3. In some cases, overlapping activities cannot be separated by observing each activity individually as is the case in patients with WPW Syndrome, where the delta wave, produced by premature ventricular excitation via the accessory pathway, merges with the end of the P wave (i.e., the repolarization of the atria).

The study of normal volunteers indicated that atrial repolarization produces a relatively stable field pattern with a decreasing amplitude during the primary portion of the P–Q interval. For this reason, the subtraction of the atrial repolarization activity from the beginning of ventricular excitation during the delta wave can be achieved in the following way: The magnetic field pattern representing the atrial repolarization is defined directly before the delta wave onset and is subsequently multiplied by a time-dependent weighting factor which serves as one of the fitting parameters in the iterative source reconstruction algorithm.

Biomagnetic imaging from single, unaveraged, heartbeats has been found to yield clinically sufficient spatial resolution, even in patients where only a single ectopic event occurred during recording. Averaging of several heartbeats, however, does improve the spatial resolution and thereby biomagnetic reconstruction during time intervals of very weak activity—such as the beginning of an extrasystole or WPW delta wave. For this reason, we applied averaging wherever more than one event was available. Two algorithms for automated detection and averaging were used: (a) an automated QRS complex detection method and (b) a correlation algorithm which automatically compares a data set with the signal of a predefined event. This is especially useful in the separation of ectopic beats from normal heartbeats in long recordings. The QRS complex which is automatically detected can be used as a trigger for averaging heart cycles. The more sophisticated correlation method uses the signal pattern of a user-defined event to automatically find other such events in a recorded data set. These can then be averaged to improve the SNR.

As previously mentioned, the imaging of bioelectric activity by means of its magnetic field assumes that the activity can be modeled as a current dipole. This assumption is valid only when the bioelectric activity is focal (concentrated in a small volume). Distributed current densities cannot unequivocally be reconstructed from their magnetic fields, which means, in the case of the heart, that biomagnetic imaging is limited to those time intervals of the heart cycle where a large muscle mass is not active (e.g., the beginning of extra systoles). Reconstruction is performed only at the time interval of interest within the heart cycle (e.g., the delta wave as shown in Fig. 4 or the onset of an ectopic beat); source location, orientation, and strength are reconstructed at each sampled data point. Due to limitations inherent in any physiological model, the validity of the reconstruction depends on the conformity of actual physiological activity and the model. The combination of the following five criteria has proven to be a powerful tool in the automated separation of valid and invalid reconstruction results:

—The deviation between the measured field map and the map produced by the reconstructed source ("goodness of fit") must not exceed a predefined threshold.
—The location of the reconstructed source must lie within anatomically defined limits, e.g., within the heart volume where MCG evaluations have been made.
—The distance to successive source locations must not exceed a value which is defined by the sampling interval and the maximum possible conductance velocity of the activated tissue.

—The location of the reconstructed source has to be stable within the aforement-ioned conductance velocity limit and within the typical duration of action or generator potentials that apply to the type of tissue under consideration.
—Where possible, upper and lower limits of the strength of the reconstructed source should be defined by electrophysiology. Furthermore, an upper limit for the rate of change of the source strength could be defined.

The end result of data evaluation is an image of the evolution of an electro-physiological process in time and space.

6 Verification of the Localization Accuracy

6.1 Phantom Studies

To investigate system performance and localization accuracy three different phantoms were studied: a single coil in air, a coil array in air, and a current dipole in a tray filled with saline solution.

Since the magnetic field of current coils can be calculated exactly, their localization provides a test of the system accuracy. The current dipole, consisting of the open ends of two threaded wires in saline solution, permits the testing of the iterative localization procedure and the validity of the infinite half-space geometry. Test procedures have been performed at various dipole/dewar distances and with the rotation of the sensor up to $40°$ in two orthogonal directions.

With coil phantoms the accuracy of localization was found to be ± 1 mm. For the current dipole in saline solution, accuracy was better than ± 2.5 mm up to a distance of 9 cm from the center of the sensor array.

6.2 Localization Accuracy Within the Human Body

6.2.1 Development of an Amagnetic Pacing Catheter

To verify the potential of biomagnetic diagnostics in the accurate localization of ectopic electrical activity in the human heart, we developed a pacing catheter that would not interfere with biomagnetic measurement but would fulfill the following criteria:

—Nonferromagnetic
—No disturbing magnetic field caused by an electric current in the feed-in wires
—Compatible with X-ray and MRI

The bipolar pacing catheter (size 5 F), which is manufactured from nonmagnetic material, carries two platinum electrodes that are placed 10 mm apart at the tip. The lead-in wires consist of a pair of twisted copper wires; the magnetic fields produced by the electric current in the lead-in wires thus neutralize each other.

In order to document the catheter position using MR tomography the catheter tip is marked with lyophilized gadolinium which causes a visible mark in the MR image.

6.2.2 Biomagnetic Localization of Paced Arrhythmias

The catheter just described was inserted via the brachial vein of healthy volunteers and stabilized within the right ventricle. The position was documented with orthogonal X-ray images in expiration. During the following 4-min biomagnetic investigation, conducted with a sampling frequency of 6 kHz, a stable ventricular rhythm was sustained by applying a stimulus of 0.8 V for 1 ms at a rate of 120/min. Each stimulus was followed by a low-voltage compensation current of 11.8 ms. After removal of the copper wires from the catheter (which was performed under fluoroscopic controle to assure that the catheter would not change its intracardial position), MR images of the thorax were acquired in three planes.

To evaluate the data, the stimuli were used as a trigger. About 100 cycles , in expiration—consisting of one stimulus and one ventricular excitation—were averaged to improve the SNR. The locus of the current dipole was reconstructed from the magnetic field distribution at the time of the stimulus by applying the iterative process described in Sect. 5 and was then projected both on the X-ray image and the MR image (Fig. 5).

As can be seen from the illustrations, the biomagnetic image of the current dipole was correctly correlated to the anatomical position of the catheter electrodes with an error of only a few mm. The small current dipole set into the myocardium was localized also 13 ms after the beginning of the pulse (0.2 ms after the end of the compensation current). The location of the current dipole about 10 mm from the tip of the catheter corresponds well to the known velocity of electrical excitation in the myocardium: about 1 mm/ms (Fig. 6).

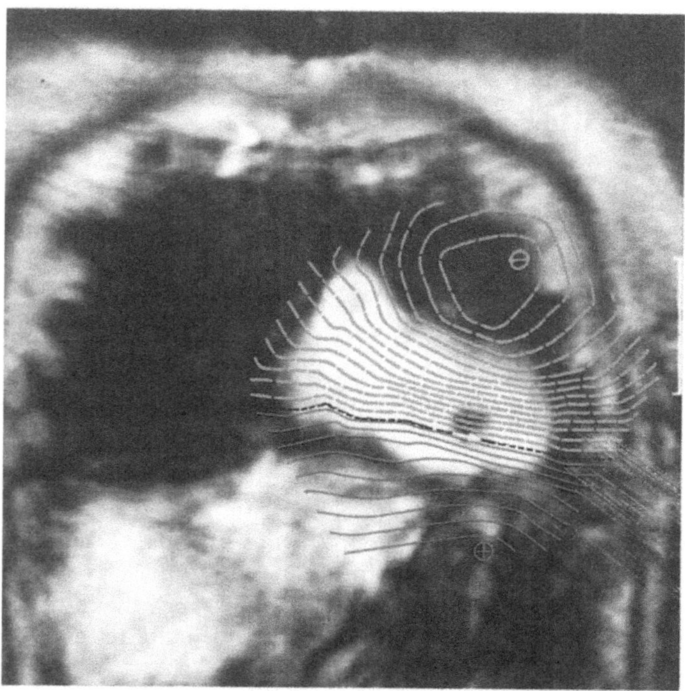

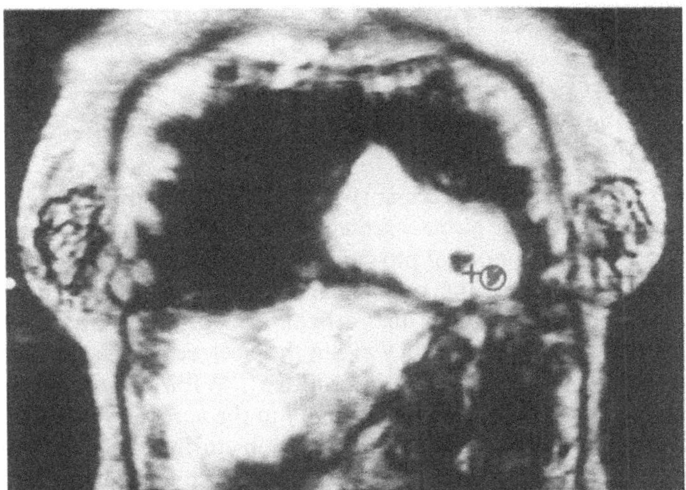

a

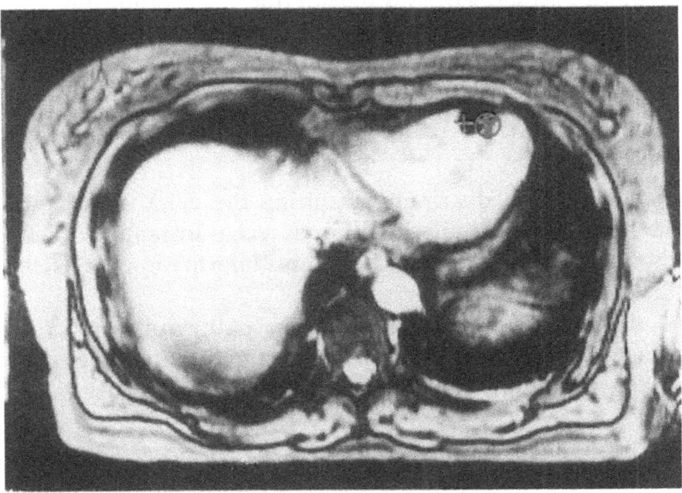

b

Fig. 6 a, b. Localization results in **a** frontal and **b** axial slices of ventricular extrasystoles provoked with a pacing catheter. The *circular disturbance* in **a** and **b** in indicates the position of the pacing catheter. The *cross* indicates the reconstructed site of the equivalent current dipole at the time of the stimulus. *The small red squares* inside the circle depict ventricular excitation 13–30 ms after the stimulus and thus onset of the extrasystole. Each *Square* represents the site of the reconstructed dipole at one time instant. The distance of about 10 mm from the stimulus corresponds well with the conduction velocity of about 1 mm/ms

◀──

Fig. 5. Magnetic field distribution during stimulus applied with pacing catheter. The *dark circular disturbance* in the MR image is caused by gadolinium in the catheter tip. The *yellow arrow* indicates the position of the electric current dipole as reconstructed from the magnetic field and projected on the MR image

7 Clinical Applications

7.1 Application to Patients with WPW Syndrome

7.1.1 Patients and Method

Patients with WPW syndrome possess accessory pathways which connect the atria and ventricles. Via these pathways, electrocardiac excitation will spread from the atria to the ventricles without the normal physiological delay of up to 200 ms. The result is a partial depolarization of the ventricular myocardium at a time when excitation should still be restricted to the atrioventricular (AV) node. This premature activity causes the so-called delta wave in the electrocardiogram. Eleven patients with symptomatic, in some cases intermittent, WPW syndrome were investigated biomagnetically and the electrical activity in the accessory conduction path was reconstructed. Following atrial depolarization during the delta wave, a series of current dipoles were localized using the magnetic field distributions. Image fusion, as previously described, allowed for the localization on an MR image.

The localization results of five patients were verified using invasive electro-physiological investigation and radionuclide ventriculography (Table 2).

7.1.2 Results

In all patients the magnetic field distributions during the delta wave could be recorded. From the magnetic field distribution at each instant in time, the equivalent current dipole was reconstructed. Using this information the excitation propagation could be visualized (Fig. 7).

In all cases, the magnetically localized accessory pathways were correctly situated in the AV plane, i.e., the area between the atria and the ventricles. In the five cases where biomagnetic findings were verfied by invasive and nuclear medicine

Table 2. Investigation of patients with WPW syndrome

Patient	Sex	Age	Localization results		
			Biomagnetic investigation	Electrophysiological mapping	Radionuclide ventriculography
H. B.	M	53	Left lateral	—	—
J. L.	F	28	Left lateral	—	—
L. B.	F	35	Left lateral	—	—
J. B.	M	22	Posteroseptal to the left	—	—
T. W.	M	26	Posteroseptal to the right	—	—
H. R.	M	38	Right free wall	—	—
R. K.	M	21	Right free wall	Right free wall	Right free wall
W. H.	M	25	Posteroseptal to the left	Posteroseptal to the left	Posteroseptal to the left
I. L.	F	44	Posteroseptal to the left	Posteroseptal to the left	Posteroseptal to the left
J. S.	F	30	Left lateral	Left lateral	Left lateral
J. Sch.	M	26	Left lateral	Left lateral	Left lateral

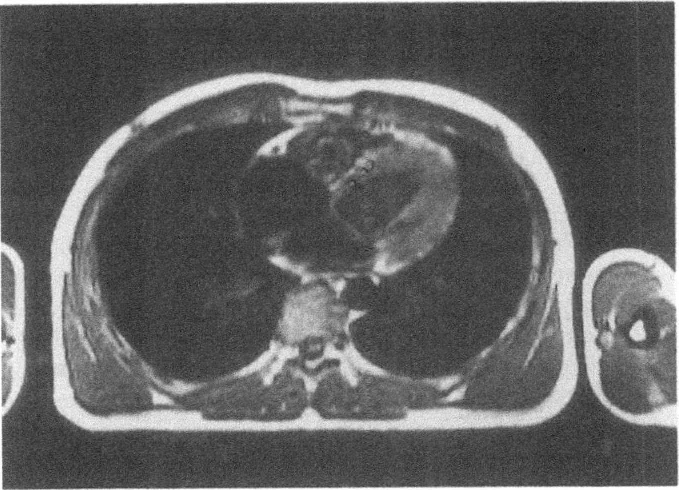

Fig. 7. Patient with WPW syndrome. Localization of accessory pathway is determined by magneto-cardiography as posteroseptal to the left. The *red squares* indicate the reconstructed site of the equivalent current dipole at every time instant over 14 ms

investigations, precise conformity was found; the results of invasive electrophysio-logical mapping corresponded to biomagnetic localization with a difference of less than 20 mm.

7.2 Application to Patients with Ventricular Extrasystoles

7.2.1 Patients and Method

In the ventricular walls of patients with ventricular extrasystoles, small areas of electrically instable myocardium cause excitation of the ventricles in addition to that normally caused by depolarization via the conductive system.

We investigated six patients where extrasystoles were caused by several different primary illnesses (Table 3). Biomagnetic data were recorded in 4–10 min examina-

Table 3. Investigation of patients with ventricular extrasystoles

Patient	Sex	Age	Clinical findings	Results of biomagnetic investigation
D. K.	F	45	Parasystole	Proximal interventricular septum
A. R.	M	47	Parasystole	Right ventricular outflow tract
U. K.	F	22	Parasystole	Apex of right ventricle
H. F.	M	42	Coronary heart disease with aneurysm of anterior wall	Septal margin of aneursym
P. H.	M	51	Coronary heart disease with aneurysm of anterior wall and apex	Anterior margin of aneursym
F. H.	M	77	Coronary heart disease with ischemia of the apical region	Apex of right ventricle

tions. Extrasystoles identified during expiration were averaged to improve the SNR; if the ventricular beat emerged from the repolarization of the preceding heart cycle, the overlapping magnetic fields were separated by applying digital subtraction as previously described (Sect. 5).

7.2.2 Results

The magnetic field distribution at the onset of ventricular ectopic heart beats permits the localization of an equivalent current dipole (Fig. 8); the intensity of the magnetic field and the strength of the reconstructed dipole increase steadily (Fig. 9). The site of origin of the ventricular extrasystole can thus be reconstructed from the magnetic field distribution during the first milliseconds of ectopic activity. The orientation of the equivalent current dipole agrees with the direction in which the excitation propagates. As the area of depolarized myocardium increases, the localized dipole increasingly represents a "summation vector" describing the complete excitation. This vector can no longer be related to a focal electric excitation (cf., Fig. 4).

Three of the six patients presented with parasystole, an illness resulting from an ectopic pacemaker in otherwise healthy myocardium. A large-scale electrophysiological investigation which was carried out in one of these cases substantially confirmed the biomegnetic finding—an ectopic focus in the proximal interventricular septum. In Fig. 10a, the dipole path depicts the excitation spreading along the interventricular septum.

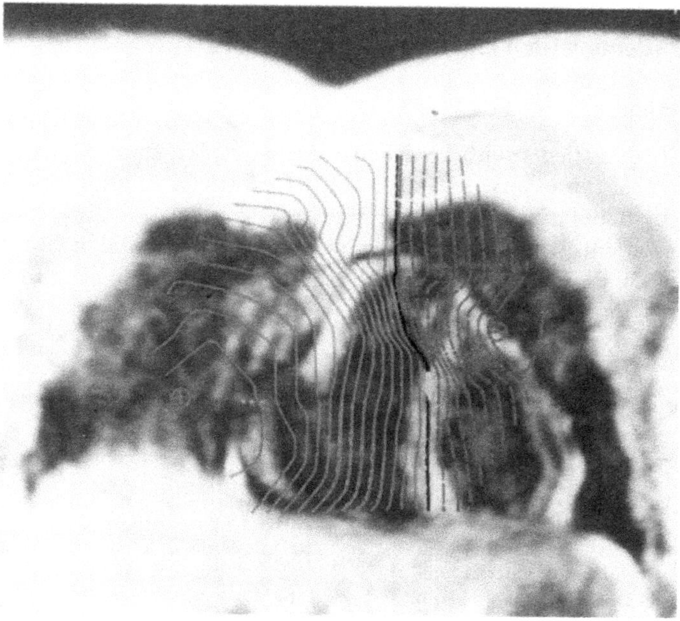

Fig. 8. Patient with parasystole. Magnetic field distribution at the onset of a single ventricular extrasystole is projected onto the MR image. The *yellow arrow* indicates the biomagnetic localization of the equivalent current dipole

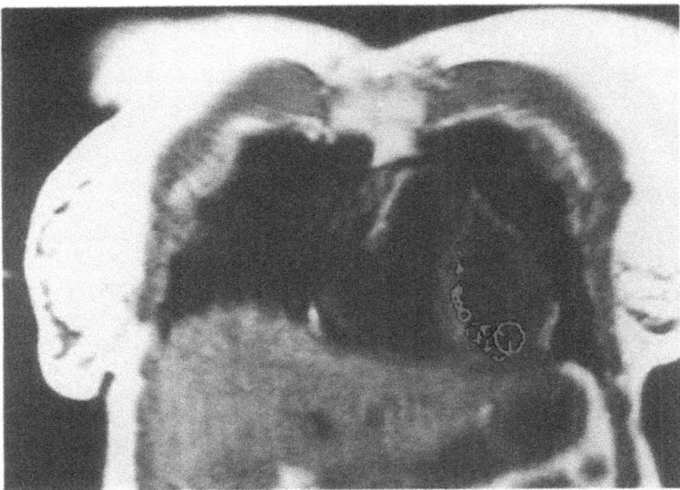

Fig. 9. Patient with parasystole. Localization results during the first 50 ms of ventricular extrasystoles (7 beats averaged). The *centers of the circles* represent the sites of the equivalent current dipoles 2 ms apart. The *diameter of the circles* represents the strength of the current dipole

Two patients presented with coronary heart disease and an aneurysm of the left ventricular wall documented in ultrasound, levocardiography, and in MRI. In both cases, the site of origin of the ectopic beat was localized at the margin of the damaged area of the myocardium (Fig. 11).

In the remaining patient, who also had coronary heart disease, the ectopic pacemaker was localized in myocardium damaged by ischemia at the apex of the right ventricle.

8 Discussion

Biomagnetic imaging makes it possible to investigate electrical processes within the human heart, without being influenced by volume currents in the tissue surrounding the source. It thus renders possible the completely noninvasive three-dimensional reconstruction of the underlying electrical activity, while localization of electric sources within the body by measurement of surface potentials remains impossible.

The precision of biomagnetic imaging so far had to be verified using indirect methods such as invasive endocardial mapping. According to certain authors, the magnetic localization of accessory pathways in patients with WPW syndrome has been found accurate to around 10 mm [5, 7, 14]. In a few cases, biomagnetic results were verified by intraoperative findings. Although difficulties in comparing these results are obvious, localization accuracy has been reported to be about 10 mm [8]. Biomagnetic localization of pacing catheters [6, 9] has also provided a means to quantify localization accuracy. Singular extrasystoles have occasionally been localized using a single channel biomagnetic system but results have not been verified. Several atrial and ventricular tachycardias were also investigated and in

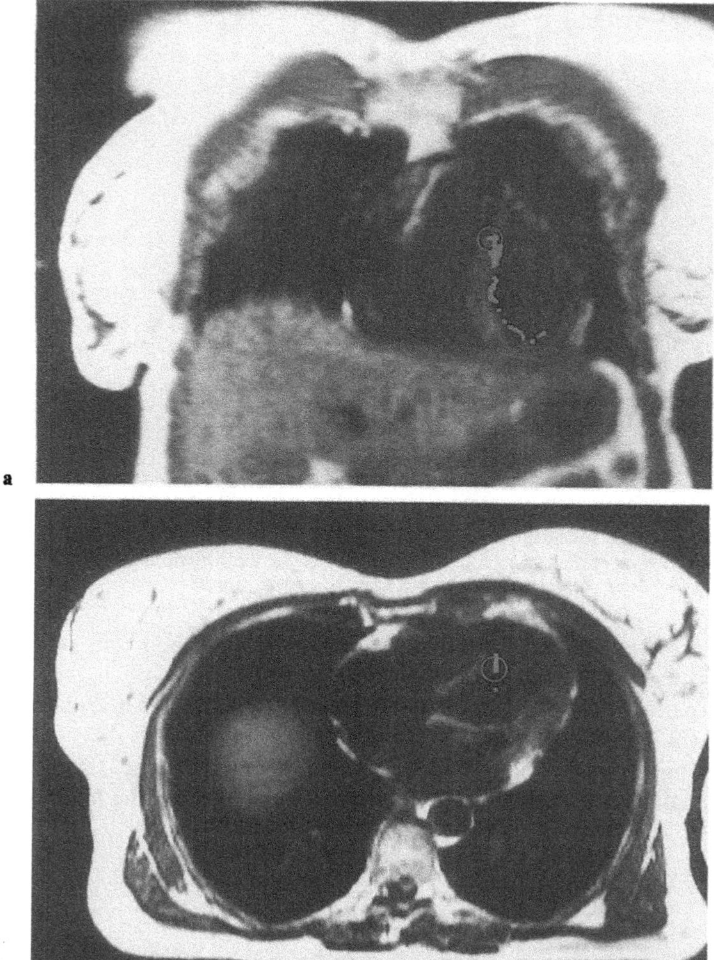

Fig. 10 a, b. Patient with parasystole. The *red squares* indicate the dipole localization during the first 50 ms of ventricular extrasystoles in **a** frontal and **b** axial projection marked in the corresponding MR image. The *circles* indicate the localization of the ectopic focus

one case the origin of a ventricular tachycardia was verified by invasive electro-physiological study [10].

The potential of biomagnetic investigations in the three-dimensional reconstruction of electrical eactivity has clearly been demonstrated in these results. However, all of these results were obtained using systems consisting of only one or a few channels that had to be adjusted for step-by-step data acquisition and the long measurement period, often lasting between 1 and 3 h, not only limited clinical application but also impaired localization accuracy.

Large-scale biomagnetic multichannel systems constitute an important step forward in biomagnetic imaging of the heart. In addition to the reduction of

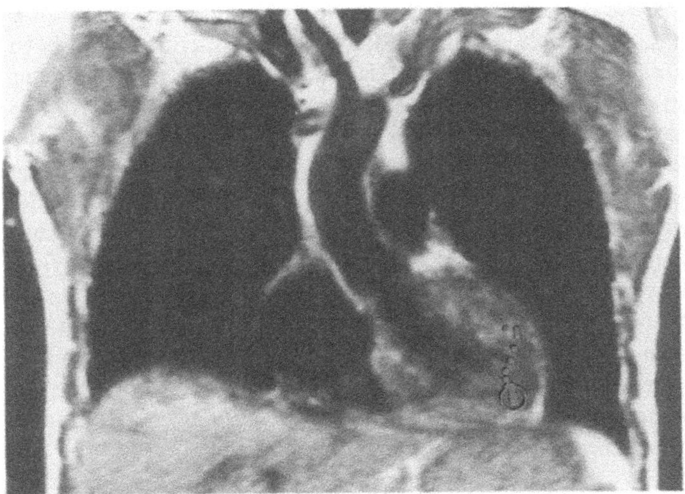

Fig. 11. Patient with coronary heart disease and aneurysm of the anterior wall and apex. The *circle* indicates the localization of the ectopic focus, situated at the margin of the aneurysm. The *red squares* depict ventricular excitation during the first milliseconds of the extrasystoles

the examination time from several hours to just a few minutes, these new systems allow coherent registration of the magnetic field and high spatial resolution with just a single adjustment of the sensors. Furthermore, rare and even singular events, such as ventricular extrasystoles, have been recorded and investigated.

Only large-scale multichannel systems permit biomagnetic imaging of electrical activity in the human heart without undue strain on the patient. This was first demonstrated in 11 patients with WPW syndrome where accessory pathways were located at various points in the heart. The results of biomagnetic imaging showed ideal correspondence to the results of other methods of investigation such as radionuclide ventriculography and invasive electrophysiological catheter mapping.

While radionuclide ventriculography on the one hand permits an approximate classification of the existing pathological condition, invasive catheter mapping allows a relatively precise determination of the site of the accessory pathways (depending on the distance between the electrodes of the catheters used). The difference in the localization results between these techniques and biomagnetic imaging has been determined to be less than 10 mm. Slight topographical differences result from the fact that the electrophysiological examination localizes the atrial insertion of the accessory pathway, whereas biomagnetic imaging and radionuclide ventriculography determine the premature beginning of ventricular muscle excitation via the accessory conduction path.

The development of our amagnetic, MR compatible, pacing catheter was essential for the direct, reproducible, verification of the spatial resolution of biomagnetic imaging. Preliminary investigations have shown that the tip of this specially designed catheter constitutes an ideal topographical reference point in X-ray and MRI. Activity resulting from the stimulus applied with the catheter, ventricular excitation provoked at a known site, and spontaneous ventricular extrasystoles showed a highly satisfactory three-demensional concordance in both MRI and biomagnetic imaging. The distance of the induced dipole from the catheter tip also provides a direct measurement of the excitation velocity in the myocardium.

The digital subtraction of disturbing underlying magnetic fields renders the application of biomagnetic imaging possible in the case of extrasystoles emerging from the repolarization of the preceding heart cycle. We applied biomagnetic imaging to patients with ventricular extrasystoles and were able to show that the ectopic electrical activity can be precisely reconstructed from the magnetic field distribution measured over the body surface.

Large-scale multichannel biomagnetic imaging represents a method that, for the first time, permits the complete noninvasive three-dimensional reconstruction and visualization of electrical phenomena in the heart. The high degree of accuracy in biomagnetic localization makes it possible to treat pathological arrhythmias surgically or using interventional catheter ablation techniques.

9 Prospects

Biomagnetic imaging of the heart for the first time permits the three-dimensional reconstruction and visualization of electromagnetic phenomena in the heart. This means that it is now possible to quickly, precisely, and noninvasively localize pathological electrical activities.

Since the annual mortality due to cardiac rhythm disorders is about 1500 per million inhabitants in industrialized nations, a simple and noninvasive means of investigating these disorders at an early stage is vital. It is only with epidemiological investigations which make widespread use of biomagnetic imaging that we can better understand and classify this inhomogeneous group of diseases and improve methods of treatment.

Biomagnetic imaging may be a key to solving a problem which has become critical for all industrial nations.

References

1. Abraham-Fuchs K, Weikl A, Schneider S, Moshage W, Röhrlein G, Wirth A, Bachmann K, Schittenhelm R (1989) Application of biomagnetic multichannel system to the comparative localization of accessory conduction pathways in patients with WPW syndrome. In: Williamson SJ, Hoke M, Stroink G, Kotani M (eds) Advances in Biomagnetism. Plenum, New York, pp 369–372
2. Baule G, McFee R (1963) Detection of the magnetic field of the heart. Am Heart J 66:95–96
3. Cohen D, Edelsack E.A, Zimmerman JE (1970) Magnetocardiograms taken inside a shielded room with a superconducting point contact magnetometer. Appl Phys Lett 16:278–280
4. Cuffin BN, Cohen D (1977) Magnetic fields of a dipole in special volume conductor shapes. IEEE Trans Biomed Eng BME 24:372–381
5. Erne SN (1985) High resolution magnetocardiography. Modelling and source localization. Med Biol Eng Comput 23 (suppl):1447–1450

6. Fenici RR, Masselli M (1986) Magnetocardiography: perspectives in clinical application. Proc of the IEEE Eng in Med and Biol Society, 8th annual conf, 1:439–440
7. Fenici RR, Masselli M, Lopez L, Melillo G (1987) Magnetocardiographic localization of arrhythmogenic tissue. 6th Int Conf Biomagn, Tokyo, pp 282–285
8. Fenici RR, Melillo G, Masselli M, Capelli A (1989) Magnetocardiographic three dimensional localization of Kent Bundles. 4th European Symposium on Cardiac Pacing, Stockholm, p 30
9. Fenici RR, Melillo G, Cappeli A, Deluca D, Masselli M (1989) Magnetocardiographic localization of a pacing catheter. 7th Int Conf Biomagn, New York, Conference Digest, pp 333–334
10. Fenici RR, Melillo G, Cappeli A, Deluca C, Masselli M (1989) Reproducibility of magneto-cardiographic imaging of arrhythmias. 7th Inf Conf Biomagn, New York, Conference Digest, pp 323–324
11. Hoenig HE, Daalmans G, Folberth W, Reichenberger H, Schneider S, Seifert H (1989) Biomagnetic multichannel system with integrated SQUIDs and first order gradiometers operating in a shielded room. Cryogenics 29:809–813
12. Kannel WB, McGee DL (1975) Epidemiology of sudden death: insights of the framingham study. In: Josephson ME (ed.) Sudden cardiac death. Davis, Philodelphia, pp 93–106
13. Kaplan MA, Cohen KL (1969) Ventricular fibrillation in the Wolff-Parkinson-White syndrome. Am J Cardiol 24:259
14. Katila T, Montonen J, Maekijaervi M, Nenonen J, Raivic M, Siltanen P (1987) Localization of the Accessory Cardiac Conduction Pathway. In: Atsumi K, Kotani M, Ueno S, et al. (eds) Biomagnetism '87. Tokyo, Tokyo Denki University Press, pp 430–433
15. Mori H, Nakaya Y (1980) Present status of clinical magnetocardiography. CV World Report 1:78–86
16. Panidis IP, Morganroth J (1985) Initiating events of sudden cardiac death. In: Josephson ME (ed) Sudden cardiac death. Davis, Philadelphia, pp 81–92
17. Surawicz B (1987) Prognosis of ventricular arrhythmias in relation to sudden cardiac death: therapeutic implications. J Am Coll Cardiol 10:2, 435–447
18. Stroink G, MacAulay CE, tenVoorde B, Montague T, Horacek BM (1986) High-resolution magnetocardiographic field mapping and analysis. 8th Conf Engl Med Biol Soc, pp 445
19. Williamson SJ, Romani GL, Kaufman L, Modena J (1982) Biomagnetism: an interdisciplinary approach. Plenum, New York

Selective Endovascular Treatment of Intracranial Aneurysms by Means of Latex Balloons Filled with a Polymerizing Substance: A Clinical and Experimental Study

M. Nonent[1,2], A. Laurent[1], A. Aymard[1], J.J. Merland[1], M. Bellet[2], J. Huguet[3], and M. Vert[3]

1 Introduction

Thanks to progress made in the area of microcatheters and balloons, it is now possible to consider endovascular treatment of intracranial aneurysms [1, 3, 7]. The ideal method consists in exclusion of the aneurysm by placing a detachable balloon inside the aneurysm pouch, while at the same time preserving the parent vessel (Fig. 1).

In order to ensure that the balloon's volume remains stable long enough to allow aneurysmal thrombosis to occur, the ballon must be inflated with a polymerizing substance which satisfies the following requirements:

1. Polymerization at 37°C.
2. High fluidity of the mixture during the procedure, allowing easy inflation and deflation of the balloon through a microcatheter.
3. Polymerization time must be precisely predicted.
4. The polymer can be mixed with hydrosoluble iodine contrast medium.
5. The polymer plug must be stable after polymerization.

[1] Service et Laboratoire de Neuroradiologie et d'Angiographie Thérapeutique, Hôpital et Faculte' Lariboisière, 2, rue Ambroise Paré 75010, Paris, France
[2] Service de Radiologie, CHU Morvan, 5 avenue Foch, F-29200 Brest, France
[3] Laboratoire des Substances Macromoléculaires, UA CNRS 500, INSA, Rouen Place Emile Blondel, BP8, 76130 Mont St. Aignan, France

Frontiers in European Radiology, Vol. 8
Eds. Baert/Heuck
© Springer-Verlag, Berlin Heidelberg 1991

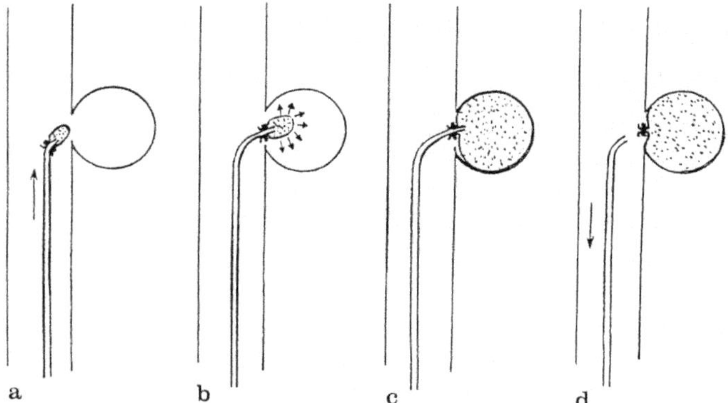

Fig. 1 A–D. Comprehensive scheme of selective endovascular treatment of intracranial aneurysms. **A** The balloon with an internal valve mechanism is brought by the microcatheter just near the aneurysm neck. **B** It is placed inside the aneurysm sack. **C** The balloon is inflated. **D** The balloon is released and the aneurysm is excluded

6. The polymer must show mechanical suppleness after polymerization.
7. Biocompatibility.
8. Ready to use.
9. Possibility of sterilization without chemical change of the mixture.

An acrylic monomer, hydroxyethylmethacrylate (HEMA), which *a priori* satisfies the main requisites, is currently being used by most interventional neuroradiology teams [2, 4, 8]. Polymerization results in a gel-like substance. The process requires that a monomer (HEMA); a cross-linking agent (ethyleneglycoldimethacrylate, EGDM) and an oxide-reducing initiator system combining ferrous ammonium sulfate (FAS) and hydrogen peroxide (H_2O_2), be mixed. The polymerization is possible because of the free radicals supplied by the initiator system. The literature reports results obtained with this polymer in silicone balloons [2, 4] commonly used in the USA, and not those obtained with latex ones; the latter are widely used in France and Europe.

The aim of this chapter which involves a follow-up analysis of seven patients, is twofold:

1. To demonstrate, by way of an experimental in vitro study, the interactions which can occur between latex and HEMA,
2. To deduce (from 1, above) the consequences for selective endovascular treatment by balloon of intracranial aneurysms.

The clinical study is deliberately restricted to the global results obtained; a complete description is intended for a future publication. In this chapter we concentrate on the experiment and its results.

2 Clinical Study

2.1 Materials and Methods

Seven patients, three men and four women, with intracranial aneurysms, (age range: 25–70; $\bar{x} = 50$) underwent treatment using detachable latex balloons, inflated with HEMA (Interventional therapeutics Corporation, ITC, San Francisco, CA, USA) at Lariboisiere Hospital between 1987 and 1989.

The aneurysms were located in three differents areas; there were three basilar trunk aneurysms, three internal carotid aneurysms (one cavernous, one supraclinoid, and one internal carotid bifurcation), and one aneurysm of the anterior communicating artery. All the patients involved in the study underwent at least one embolization; a total of ten embolizations were carried out. A 1-French polyethylene microcatheter (Balt, Montmorency, France; inner diameter: 0.2 mm, outer diameter: 0.33 mm) was used carrying a latex balloon with an internal valve. It was released using the coaxial technique previously described and perfected by *Merland* and *Ruffenacht* [6]. The balloon was released only when it was certain that the HEMA had been polymerized; a check sample was used to confirm this. The polymerization time was 40–60 min. Follow-up was judged by plain radiographs (evolution of X-ray opacity of the balloon), angiography (exclusion of the aneurysm), and/or MRI (aneurysmal thrombosis, intrasaccular flow). The average follow-up period was 9 months, although one patient died 5 days after embolization.

2.2 Results

Angiographic investigations carried out immediately after embolization showed nine complete occlusions and one subtotal occlusion of the aneurysm. Three aneurysm exclusions were obtained conclusively, once without complication, once with stenosis of an anterior cerebral artery of no serious clinical signifiance, and once with stenosis of a middle cerebral artery responsible for a non-regressive stroke.

Five aneurysm repermeations were observed. Four of these were early repermeations (angiographic findings 1–5 months after embolization), of which three were in the same patient, who had a large aneurysm of the right supraclinoid internal carotid artery. The fifth was a late repermeation observed 2 years after embolization in a female patient who had only had an initial partial occlusion.

One arterial occlusion occurred 5 days after the treatment of an aneurysm of the tip of the basilar artery. The X-ray results showed the balloon split in two, with the polymer appearing to be inhomogeneous and with a partial loss of its X-ray opacity. The lower fragment of the broken balloon, filled with polymer, moved out of the aneurysmal pouch, occluding the basilar trunk. This had very serious clinical consequences (brainstem edema, coma).

One patient with an aneurysm of the basilar trunk bifurcation died on the 5th day of a stroke subsequent to a bilateral squeezed stenosis on both right and left posterior cerebral arteries.

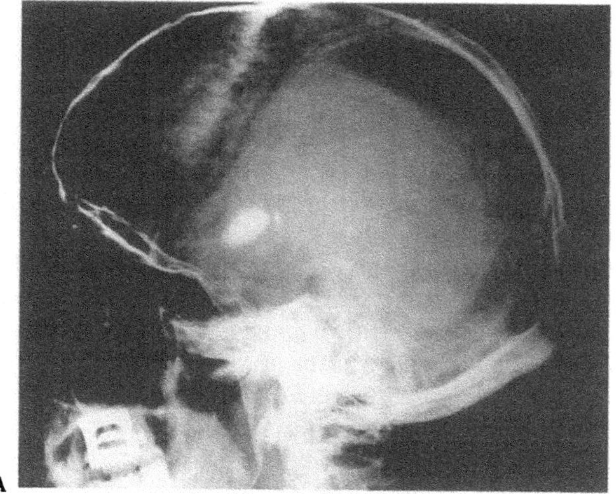

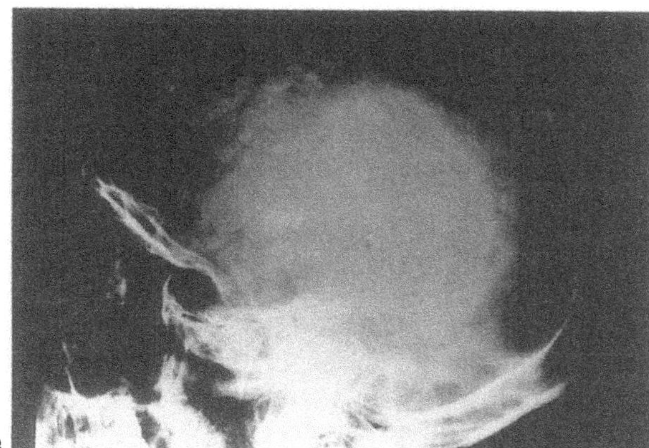

Fig. 2 A, B. In vivo X-ray evolution of a latex balloon filled with HEMA. The balloon placed inside a right supraclinoid carotid aneurysm looses its opacity. Plain radiograph immediately after embolization (**A**) and 3 weeks later (**B**)

Of ten embolizations, nine early losses of X-ray opacity in the balloons were observed within 1 month (Fig. 2).

3 In Vitro Experimental Study

The question under consideration is whether the repermeations can be linked to the loss of X-ray opacity, in other words, whether a loss of the contrast medium results in a loss of volume of the polymer. The loss of X-ray opacity could, in stead be linked to a defect in the permeability of the latex balloons or to balloon deterioration resulting in the diffusion of the contrast media out of the gel.

3.1 Materials and Methods

Six valve balloons (Table 1 and Fig. 3) were released in a normal saline and were kept at 37°C.

Five balloons, three latex and two silicone, were inflated with one of two commercially available HEMA mixtures made opaque using an iodine contrast medium. Low osmolar contrast medium (LOCM) used was either a hyper-osmolar contrast medium (iopamidol, 300 mg I/ml (Iopamiron, Schering, Lys-Lez-Lannoy, France) or an iso-osmolar contrast medium (metrizamide, 180 mg I/ml (Amipaque*, Winthrop, Clichy, France). The amount of contrast material in the polymerizing mixtures was 30% or 50%.

The essential difference between the two HEMA preparations is in the use of 30% hydrogen peroxide in the HEMA Polymerane and 3% hydrogen peroxide in the HEMA ITC. Use of 30% hydrogen peroxide reduces the hydric concentration in the gel and the final substance is thus more firm.

One latex balloon (Elastotechnics, Paris, France) was inflated using only iopamidol, with a mixture of FAS and 3% hydrogen peroxide in proportions similar to those used to obtain polymerization of HEMA.

Table 1. In vitro experimental study: characteristics of balloons used

Type of balloon	Contents[a]	Intital volume (ml)
No. 1, silicone	HEMA/metrizamide 180 mg/ml	0.45
No. 2, latex	HEMA/metrizamide 180 mg/ml	0.7
No. 3, latex	Mélange iopamidol, FAS, H_2O_2	0.7
No. 4, silicone	HEMA/iopamidol 300 mg/ml	0.6
No. 5, latex	HEMA/iopamidol 300 mg/ml	0.7
No. 6, latex	Polymerane/iopamidol 300 mg/ml	0.7

[a] The specific drugs used were Amipaque (metrizamide) and Iopamiron 300 (iopamidol)

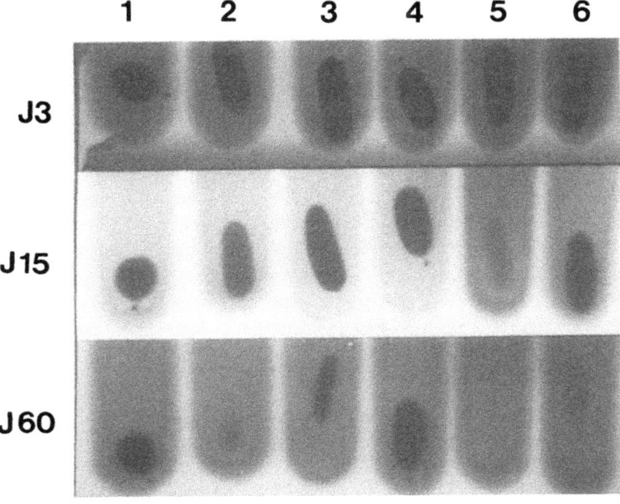

Fig. 3. In vitro X-ray evolution of latex and silicone balloons on days. 3, 15 and 60. The balloons (with the exception of balloon no. 3, see Table 2) are filled with HEMA. Balloons which are still inflated and X-ray opaque on day 60 are silicone balloons

The balloons were closely observed for 60 days so that the follow-up of X-ray opacity could be monitored. The study of latex in infrared spectrophotometry (1760 Infrared Fourier Transform Spectrometer, Perkin Elmer Norwalk, CT, USA) allowed us to analyze the chemical changes brought about by the oxide-reducing system and by the polymerizing HEMA.

3.2 Results

Table 2 shows the variations in volume of the in vitro balloons observed over a period of 60 days. Figure 3 illustrates the evolution of X-ray opacity in the balloons on days 3, 15 and 60, after inflation and releasing. All the latex balloons inflated

Table 2. Volume of balloons: follow-up results

	Day 7 (%)	Day 20 (%)	Day 60 (%)
1S HEMA, métrizamide	+6	−1.8	−11.1
2L HEMA, métrizamide	−4.8	−15	−33
3L Iopamidol, H_2O_2, FAS	+11.9	+0.1	Total deflation
4A HEMA, Iopamidol	+13	+24.9	+31.7
5L HEMA, iopamidol	+19	−25	−40
6L Polymerane, iopamidol	+6.1	+20.3	−2

S, silicone; L, latex

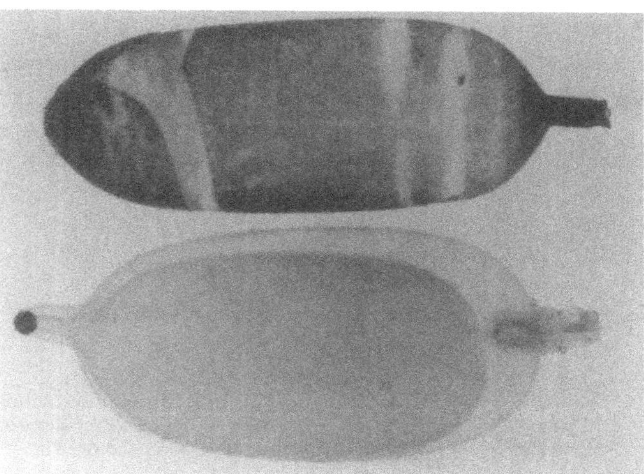

Fig. 4. Comparison between a latex balloon (upper) and a silicone balloon (*lower*) filled with HEMA and released 8 months previously in normal saline at 37°C. The splits of latex occurred during the first days after inflation, and the swelling of the sillicone balloon by osmotic mechanism are well seen. A hydric layer is obvious between the silicone wall and the gel

with HEMA (ITC or Polymerane) showed obvious evidence of deterioration (Fig. 4) with fractures in the latex visible generally from the first few days onwards (day 5 for balloon no. 5, day 9 for balloon no. 6, and day 20 for balloon no. 2). This deterioration is associated with an early loss of X-ray opacity. The silicone balloons were still X-ray opaque on the 60th day and showed no signs of damage (Fig. 4). Balloon no. 3, inflated with iopamidol and a mixture of FAS and hydrogen peroxide, lost its shape became soft and porous, and as a result deflated. The latex was not ruptured.

4 Discussion

Whichever from of HEMA is used, latex balloons show early deterioration which results in a continuous diffusion of the contrast material out of the gel. The consequences of this are: Early loss of both in vivo and in vitro X-ray opacity and varying loss of volume. With HEMA, which has a slight initial hydric concentration (Polymerane) this loss of volume can be limited to 2% for 2 months. However, a more serious loss of volume occurs with HEMA ITC, which has a higher hydric concentration. Our explanation for this is that the Polymerane compensates for the loss of the contrast medium by tending to become hydrated.

This loss of volume results in early repermeations of aneurysms in vivo. The late repermeation we observed cannot be directly attributed to this volume loss because the occlusion of the pouch was never total and, as is well known, the results in that case are never satisfactory [5]. When the HEMA is not perfectly homogeneous inside the balloon, the latex rupture becomes a dramatic event. In that case, the polymer which is still viscous, but not hard, can move out of the aneurysm pouch and occlude the parent artery. Our observation of the occlusion of the basilar trunk unfortunately leaves no doubt of this.

The chemical mechanisms in the deterioration of latex account for the fact that no HEMA mixture currently available is satisfactory. Free radicals given by initiator system allow polymerization of HEMA. Those free radicals result in a split in the residual double bonds ($C=C$), necessarily present in natural latex. Comparative infrared spectrophotometric studies of intact latex with deteriorated latex provide conclusive proof of this hypothesis: the sizeable peak at $1730\,cm^{-1}$ corresponds to the carbonyl ($C=O$) bonds (outcome of the oxidation of the $C=C$ bonds).

Thus the initiator system used to obtain HEMA polymerization does oxidize the latex HEMA aggravates the deterioration of the latex: it can be chemically grafted on latex after the double bonds ($C=C$) are opened by the free radicals of the oxidoreducing system.

In practice this oxidation results in a loss of mechanical characteristics of balloon elasticity and a weakening which leads to rupture.

Silicone balloons have already been used with HEMA in the USA for many years. American studies note the lack of intereaction between silicone and HEMA [2]. Our study confirms the absence of in vitro deterioration of silicone balloons

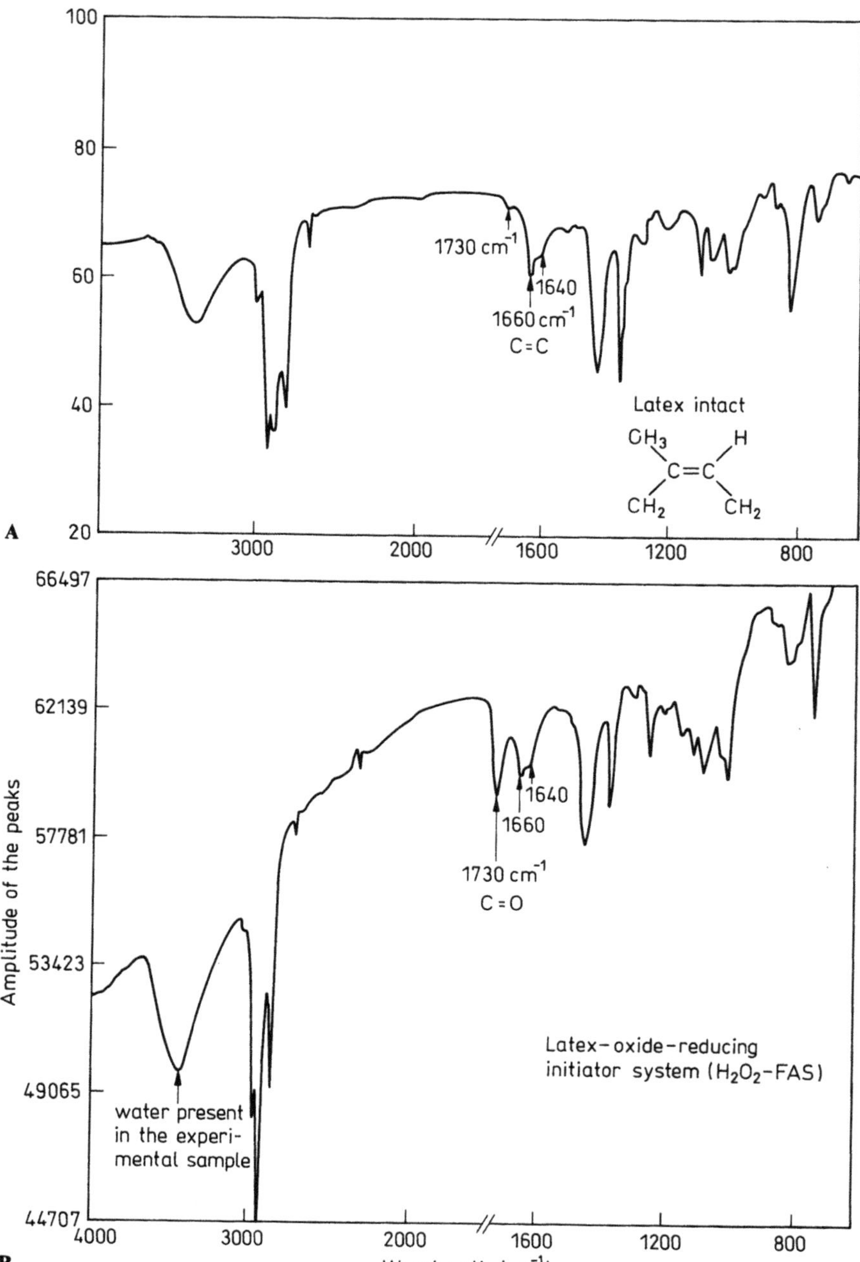
100
80
60
40
20
A
1730 cm⁻¹
1640
1660 cm⁻¹
C=C
Latex intact
CH₃
H
C=C
CH₂
CH₂
3000
2000
1600
1200
800
66497
62139
57781
53423
49065
44707
Amplitude of the peaks
1640
1660
1730 cm⁻¹
C=O
Latex-oxide-reducing
initiator system (H₂O₂-FAS)
water present
in the experi-
mental sample
4000
3000
2000
1600
1200
800
B
Wavelength (cm⁻¹)

which are inflated with HEMA. Silicone balloons are chemically inert, without any double bond (C=C), and are therefore unaffected by oxidating agents.

On the other hand, the variations in volume which occur in silicone balloons are due to the osmolality of the contrast media used and are linked to the semipermeable nature of these balloons, already referred to in scientific papers [2, 3].

In order that the volume in silicone balloons remains stable, *Hieshima* recommends the use of a very slightly hyperosmolar contrast medium, such as metrizamide, 220 mgI/ml [3]. This is in keeping with the findings of our study.

5 Conclusion

For selective embolization of intracranial aneurysms there are thus two current possibilities.

One can either continue to use latex balloons with HEMA because these balloons have the advantage of being quite remarkably elastic. Use of a concentrated HEMA preparation which will maintain its volume is advocated in this case. The latex will deteriorate very early on. The perfect homogeneity of the mixture inside the balloon must thus be assured. The other option is to use silicone balloons which are chemically stable but have the disadvantages of poor elasticity and excessive semi-permeability.

These solutions must be examined in the light of long-term results obtained by different research teams. At the same time the possibility of other solutions must not be discounted. Thus basic research in this field must be continued in order to develop a perfect polymer/balloon system and to evaluate others methods of treatment such as the use of endovascular microcoils.

6 Summary

Permanent selective exclusion by detachable balloons with parent vessel perservation is considered to be the endovascular treatment of choice of intracranial aneurysms. It has been proposed that replacement of contrast material within the balloon with a polymerizing substance will eliminate balloon deflation. Despite this solution, our clinical experience with latex balloons show that deflation can occur when balloon filling material is polyhydroxyethylmethacrylate (HEMA). We present experimental work demonstrating the chemical incompatibility between HEMA and latex. The resulting degradation of latex explains balloon deflation. Comparative in vitro results with silicone balloons are reported.

Fig. 5 A, B. Comparative infrared spectrum of **A** a referential intact latex, and **B** a latex which has been in contact with a mixture of ferrous ammonium sulfate and hydrogen peroxide (in the proportions used to obtain polymerization of HEMA). In **B** a significative peak appears at 1730 cm^{-1} (*large arrow*) which is the specific infrared wave length of carbonyl bonds (C = 0). The latex has undergone oxidation

Acknowledgements. Many thanks to Miss C. Baudot and Miss S. Fauquet for their contribution to experimental works, and to Mrs A. McKillop who helped us to translate this paper from French into English.

References

1. Debrun G, Lacour P, Caron JP, Hurth M, Comoy J, Keravel Y, (1978) Detachable Balloon and calibrated-leak balloon techniques in the treatment of cerebral vascular lesions. J Neurosur 49:635–649
2. Goto K, Halbach VV, Hardin CW, Higashida RT, Hieshima GB (1988) Permanent inflation of detachable balloons with a low-viscosity hydrophilic polymerizing system. Radiology 169:787–790
3. Hieshima GB, Grinnel VS, Mehringer CM (1987) A detachable balloon for therapeutic transcatheter occlusions. Radiology 138:227–228
4. Hieshima .B, Higashida RT, Halbach VV, Cahan L, Goto K (1986) Intravascular balloon embolization of a carotid-ophtalmic artery aneurysm with preservation of the parent vessel. AJNR 7:916–918
5. Higashida RD, Halbach VV, Cahan LD, Hieshima GB, Konishi Y. (1989) Detachable balloon embolization therapy of posterior circulation intracranial aneurysms. J, Neurosur 71:512–519
6. Merland JJ, Ruffenacht D (1985) A detachable latex balloon with valve mechanism for the permanent occlusion of large brain arterio-venous fistulas or cerebral arteries. Valk J (ed) Neuroradiology. Elsevier Amsterdam Science Publ PV, (1974)
7. Serbinenko FA (1974) Balloon catheterization and occlusion of major cerebral vessels. J Neurosurg 41:125–145
8. Taki W, Handa H, Yamagata S, Ishikawa M, Iwata H, Ikada Y (1980) Radioopaque solidifying liquids for releasable balloon technique. A technical not. Surg Neurol 13:140–142

Self-Expandable Endoprostheses as an Adjunct to Balloon Angioplasty in the Treatment of Peripheral Arterial Lesions

D. Vorwerk and R.W. Günther

1 Introduction

Since Charles Dotter first published his idea of percutaneous insertion of an intravascular endoprosthesis as an adjunct to balloon angioplasty in 1969 [3], numerous types of vascular stents have been described in the radiological literature, and some have already become a clinically important advanced technique in the treatment of vascular occlusive disease [7, 13, 19]. Active or passive expansion are employed as two different principles for increasing the diameter of the endoprosthesis once inserted into the vessel. Some stents are self-expanding using the memory effect of nitinol wire as those devices published by *Cragg* and *Rabkin* [5, 15]. Self-expanding endoprostheses utilizing the spring-coil characteristics of stainless steel wire have been described with the Gianturco–Wallace zig zag stent, the Maass spiral, and the Wallstent [10, 19, 22]. Other devices, such as the Palmaz device and the Strecker endoprosthesis, are passively expanded by a balloon [12, 20]. Clinical application of vascular stenting necessitates development of a safe delivery system which allows exact placement of the endoprosthesis used. These problems have been sufficiently overcome for the Wallstent, the Palmaz device, the Strecker endoprosthesis, and the Gianturco–Wallace stent.

Department of Diagnostic Radiology, Technical University of Aachen, W-5100 Aachen, FRG

Frontiers in European Radiology, Vol. 8
Eds. Baert/Heuck
© Springer-Verlag, Berlin Heidelberg 1991

Furthermore, a stent is characterized by its mechanical properties, which include flexibility, elasticity and radial force. The Palmaz device and the Gianturco-Wallace stent are rigid and nonelastic and have a high radial force. Both the Strecker stent and the Wallstent are flexible, but the Strecker stent, being nonelastic, has a rather low radial force. The Wallstent, however, is both flexible and elastic and is provided with a relatively high radial force. Although the mechanical characteristics of the different devices result from their particular construction principles rather than from biological requirements, obvious differences in clinical applicability have not yet been proved between the different devices [7, 13].

We describe our experiences with the self-expandable Wallstent in the peripheral arterial system since 1987.

2 Materials and Methods

2.1 The Self-Expandable Wallstent

The Wallstent prosthesis (Medivent Inc. Lausanne, and Schneider Inc. Zurich, Switzerland) is a tubular structure braided from surgical grade spring stainless steel monofilaments. Because of the spring characteristics of the monofilaments, and because the braided elements are free to pivot over each other, the prosthesis can be elastically stretched to an elongated format of small diameter. When released, the stent will recoil to its shorter, preset, unconstrained diameter. The unconstrained diameters of the stent is selected so as to be between 1 and 2 mm larger than the target vessel. When implanted, the stent can then exert a residual radial pressure against the vessel wall, preventing collapse and holding the stent in place. The stent is premounted on a flexible delivery catheter, permitting passage of tortuous vessels (Fig. 1a). The distal catheter segment remains flexible despite the presence of the mounted prosthesis. The maximum external diameters of the delivery device employed were 7 french for stents of 7–10 mm unconstrained diameters and 9 french for 12–14 mm unconstrained diameters. The catheter is coaxial, the inner shaft being joined to the external shaft by an invaginated tubular rolling membrane, which covers and retains the stent stretched on the inner shaft. Hydraulic pressure of 3.5–4 atm (350–400 kPa) applied to the annular space between the two layers of the rolling membrane facilitates withdrawal of the membrane. Peeling the membrane back like an inverted glove (Fig. 1b, c), therefore, allows the constrained prosthesis to open progressively. As long as the stent is only partially deployed, it can be retrieved toward the puncture site by pulling out the delivery system. In order to avoid inadvertent further deployment of the stent during this maneuver, the hydraulic pressure has to be released. Pushing the partially open stent will not result in repositioning but must be avoided because the open end will engage the vessel wall. Complete coverage of the lesion by the stent has to be provided. In case an ostial lesion such as at the aortic bifurcation

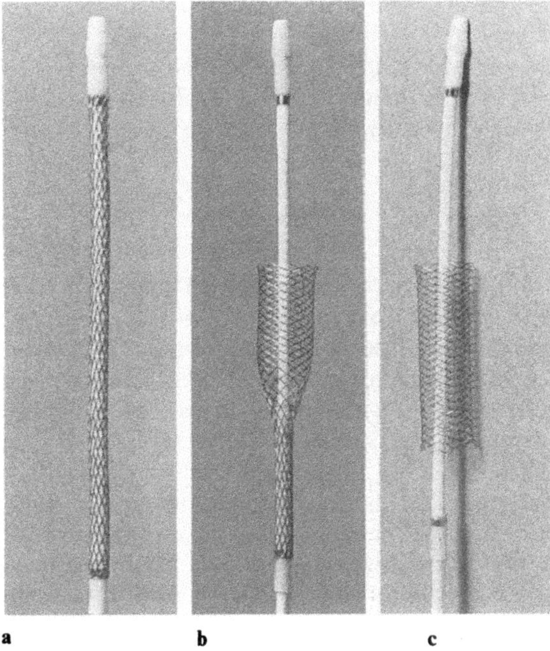

a   b   c

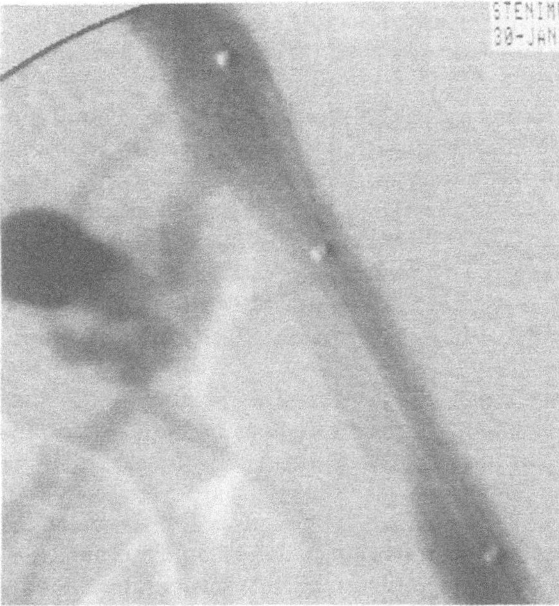

d

Fig. 1 a–d. Self-expandable
Wallstent. a The stretched stent
is premounted on a catheter
and fixed by a double layer
membrane. b By pulling back
the rolling membrane the stent
is progressively deployed.
c Stent is set free by complete
withdrawal of the outer
membrane. d Opening of the
stent within the vessel
monitored by DSA

is treated, slight protrusion of the proximal end of the prosthesis into the aorta will help to keep the iliac orifice open.

During deployment of the endoprosthesis, its position can be monitored by fluoroscopy. Because of the low visibility of the device, digital subtraction angiography (Fig. 1d) is frequently helpful in identifying the stent structure in obese patients or bowel gas superposition.

2.2 Patients

A total of 123 patients (21 women and 102 men) ranging in age from 36 to 73 years ($\bar{x} = 55.8$) were treated. All patients suffered from clinical symptoms of arterial occlusive disease. Eight patients had stage IIa disease (walking distance 200 m and more), 108 patients had stage IIb (walking distance less than 200 m). Four patients presented with pain at rest (stage III) and three with cutaneous necrosis (stage IV). The lesions were situated in the common iliac artery ($n = 67$), the external iliac artery ($n = 25$) or both of these arteries ($n = 11$). Forty-eight iliac stenoses with a mean length of 3.1 cm (range 0.5–8.0 cm) and 55 iliac occlusions with a mean length of 5.5 cm (range 1–22 cm) were stented. In 20 patients, a lesion of the superficial femoral artery was treated. The length of femoral occlusions ($n = 13$) ranged from 2 to 14 cm ($\bar{x} = 6.8$ cm), and the length of femoral stenoses ($n = 7$) from 2 to 27 cm ($\bar{x} = 5.4$ cm).

A total of 172 vascular endoprostheses were used. The implanted length of the single stents ranged from 20 mm to 75 mm. In case a lesion extended the length of a single stent, more than one device was implanted, with an overlap. Some 85 patients received one, 31 got 2 and 7 patients got 3 or more implants. The expanded diameters of the endoprostheses varied between 6 and 14 mm. The preferred diameters were: 6–7 mm for femoral implants, 8–10 mm for the external iliac artery, 10–14 mm for the common iliac artery.

Preoperative medication, of 500 mg aspirin 24 h prior to the procedure and 100–500 mg aspirin on the day of the procedure, was administered. An intraoperative dose of 5000 IU heparin was given; this was supplemented by a further 2000 IU if the procedure took more than 1 h. The protocol included postoperative heparinization for 24 h at a rate of 1000 IU/h for iliac stents and a continued daily medication of aspirin (100–500 mg). For femoral lesions, a postprocedural anticoagulation by warfarin for 3–6 months after treatment was used in 14 of 20 patients. The remaining six patients underwent a postprocedural heparinization (1000 IU/h) for 72 h.

In the early phase of the study, a limited number of iliac patients who had either a pretreatment occlusion or outflow problems, such as an occlusion of the ipsilateral superficial femoral artery, also underwent short-term anticoagulation after treatment. Because of the convincing results of iliac stenting, even in patients with outflow problems, this concept was soon abandoned. Before being discharged, all patients underwent a postoperative clinical and Doppler evaluation, while intravenous digital subtraction angiography (i.v. DSA) was performed only occasionally. The follow-up protocol included angiographic control of all patients exhibiting symptomatology as well as clinical and i.v. DSA studies at 1 or 3, and

6 and 12 months. In cases where the follow-up period exceeded 12 months, additional controls were performed at 6 or 12 month intervals.

2.3 Indications for Stent Placement

Generally, patients were considered for stent treatment only if their lesions were thought to represent a relatively high risk of failure for conventional angioplasty

Table 1. Morphology of iliac lesions

	Lesions	
Type	No.	No. of Patients
Occlusions		55
Stenoses		48
Eccentric lesion	20	
Ulcerated plaque or aneurysm	10	
Collapsing stenosis	12	
Ostial lesion	8	
Restenosis	7	
Long-segment stenosis	6	
Flow-impairing dissection	8	

(combined characters possible)

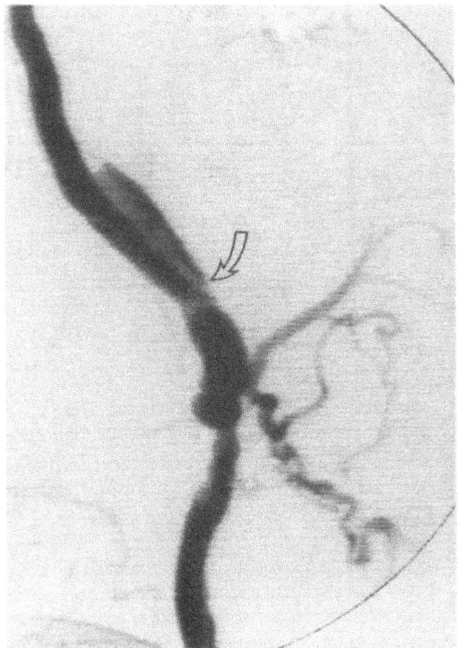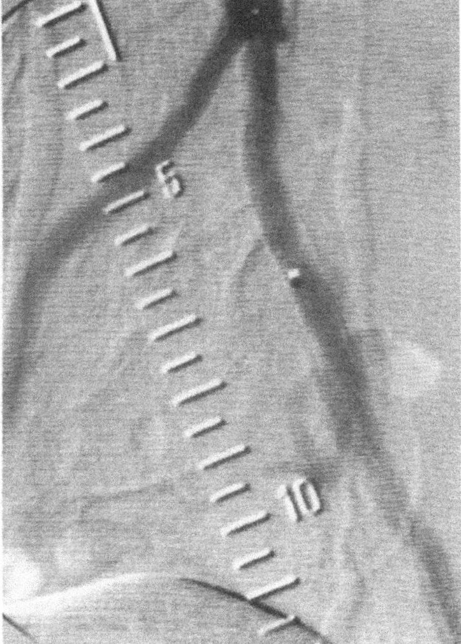

Fig. 2a, b. Stenting of a postangioplasty dissection. a Flow-relevant dissection of the common iliac artery after PTA (*arrow*). b Following stent implantation a fully restored lumen is seen

with respect to either immediate technical success or the long-term result. Neither for iliac stenoses nor femoral lesions in general was there an absolute indication for stenting, and it was performed only after state-of-the-art balloon angioplasty had yielded an insufficient result.

In iliac stenoses, eccentric lesions (recoiling or highly irregular stenoses) with ulcerative plaques or aneurysmal formation were frequent reasons for stent placement (Table 1). Furthermore, ostial lesions, long-segment stenoses, or flow-obstructing dissections (Fig. 2) after balloon dilatation, led to subsequent stent implantation. In most patients a combination of those patterns was found (Table 1) In contrast, stent placement of iliac occlusions older than 4 months was performed as a primary procedure prior to complete balloon angioplasty. After careful balloon dilatation with small balloons of 5–6 mm in diameter, a small working channel was created for stent placement (Fig. 3). Thus, a suitable endoprosthesis was implanted in the occluding segment and was redilated in case it did not open completely to its predetermined size.

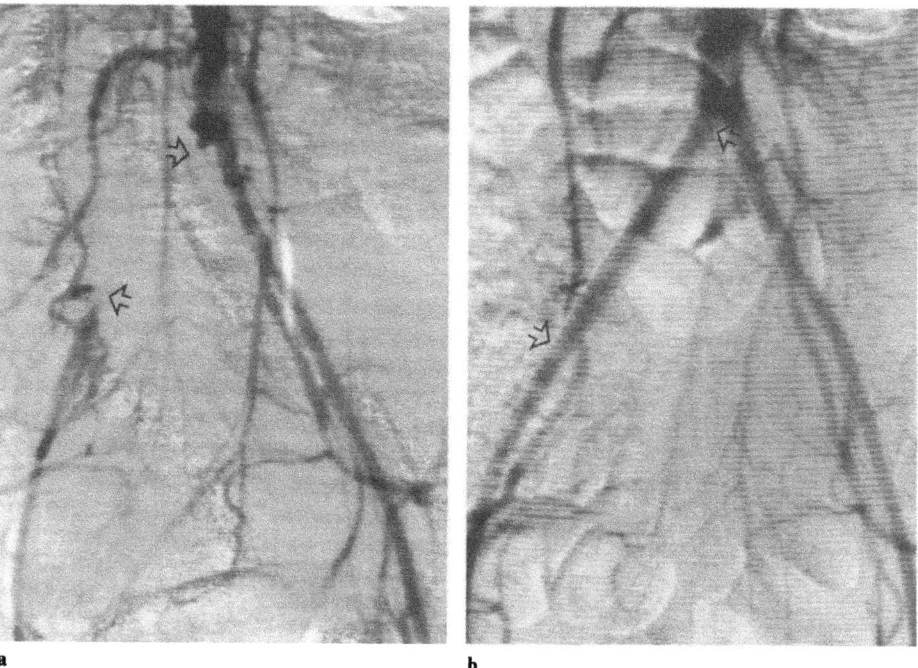

a   b

Fig. 3a, b. Iliac occlusion. **a** Completely occluded right common iliac artery (*open arrows*) in a young female patient with stroke. **b** After stent implantation the vessel is completely revascularized (*open arrows*)

3 Results

3.1 Technical Success

Primary technical success was achieved in 121 of 123 patients. In two patients with femoral implants early thrombosis occurred within 24 to 72 h after treatment. One of them was successfully treated by thrombolysis and short-term anticoagulation; the other showed a repeat reocclusion despite warfarin therapy. Additional complications occurred in 12 patients (Table 2). Three patients with

Table 2. Treatment of 12 patients exhibiting complications

Complication	Lesion		Treatment		
	Iliac (n = 103)	Femoral (n = 20)	Surgical (n = 123)	Percutaneous (n = 123)	No/conservative (n = 123)
Acute thrombosis	0	2	0	2	0
Transient embolism	0	3	0	0	3
Contralateral embolism	2	0	1	1	0
Ipsilateral embolism	1	0	0	0	1
Aortic dissection	1	0	0	0	1
Large groin hematoma	0	2	2	0	0
Septicemia	1	0	0	0	1
Total	5 (4.9%)	7 (35%)	3 (2.4%)	3 (2.4%)	6 (4.9%)

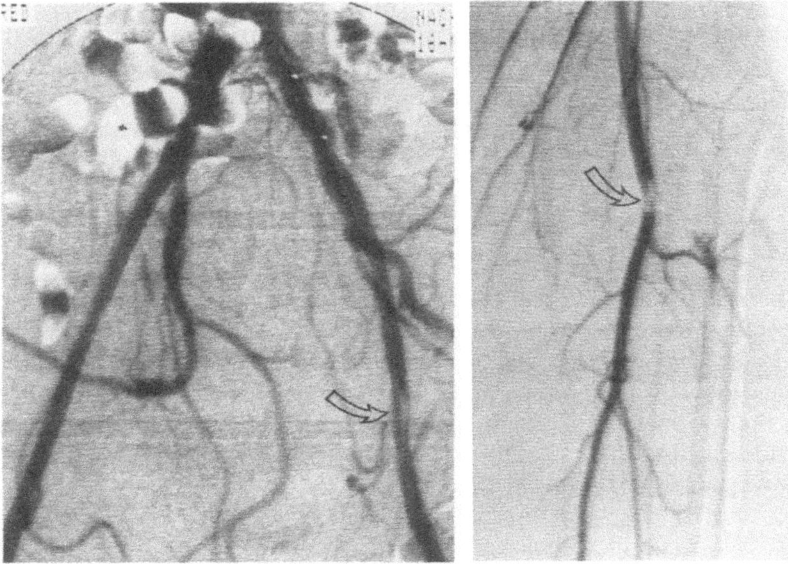

Fig. 4 a, b. Embolic complication. **a** After revascularization of a complete obstruction of the left external iliac artery, the distal end was not completely covered by the stent. Note embolus (*arrow*). **b** Dislodgement of the embolus to the popliteal artery, which lysed spontaneously under heparin infusion

Table 3. Clinical stages of arterial occlusive disease before and after treatment

Fontaine's stage	Iliac lesions		Femoral lesions	
	Before	After	Before	After
I	0	77	0	18
IIa	8	23	0	0
IIb	89	3	19	1
III	4	0	0	0
IV	2	0	1	1

femoral stents showed episodic claudications within the first week, indicating transient embolism. Manifest embolism of occluding thrombotic material with ipsilateral ($n = 1$) or contralateral ($n = 2$) dislodgement occurred in three patients treated for iliac occlusions (Fig. 4). Surgical or percutaneous intervention was necessary in only 6 of the 12 patients. Relative incidence of complications was much higher in patients treated for femoral than for iliac lesions.

3.2 Early Results

At 3-month follow-up the mean anrle/arm index of iliac patients was increased from 0.54 to 0.90. Two patients were symptomatic again because of a reobstruction of the stented segment. Clinically, the majority of patients improved for one or two stages (Table 3). One patient with a previous stage IV presented with stage IIb after treatment and two patients with early reobstruction remained in stage IIb.

For femoral lesions, the mean ankle/arm index improved from 0.6 to 0.95 3 months after treatment. Eighteen of 20 patients showed a clinically relevant improvement in their walking distances (Table 3). One patient remained in stage IV, another in stage IIb. No reocclusion or restenosis occurred within the first 3 months.

3.3 Follow-up

Follow-up time was 2–37 months ($\bar{x} = 16.5$ months). Seventeen patients were followed up for 24 and more months, and 67 for 12–23 months; 32 lesions were followed up for 6–11 months, while 7 were followed up for less than 6 months. Surgical removal of the stent was performed for two implants during aortobifemoral bypass for the treatment of an aortic aneurysm. One patient died 16 months after treatment unrelated to the procedure. Clinically, no recurrence or worsening of symptoms was found in 93 of 101 iliac patients during a follow-up exceeding 3

Fig. 5 a, d. Femoral occlusion. **a** Complete occlusion of the right superficial femoral artery. **b** Immediately after stent implantation a smoothly outlined vessel is visible. **c** After 6 months, multiple stenoses caused by intimal hyperplasia (*arrows*) were revealed within the stent leading to recurrent symptoms. **d** Atherectomy using an 8F system leads to a smoothly outlined inner stent surface

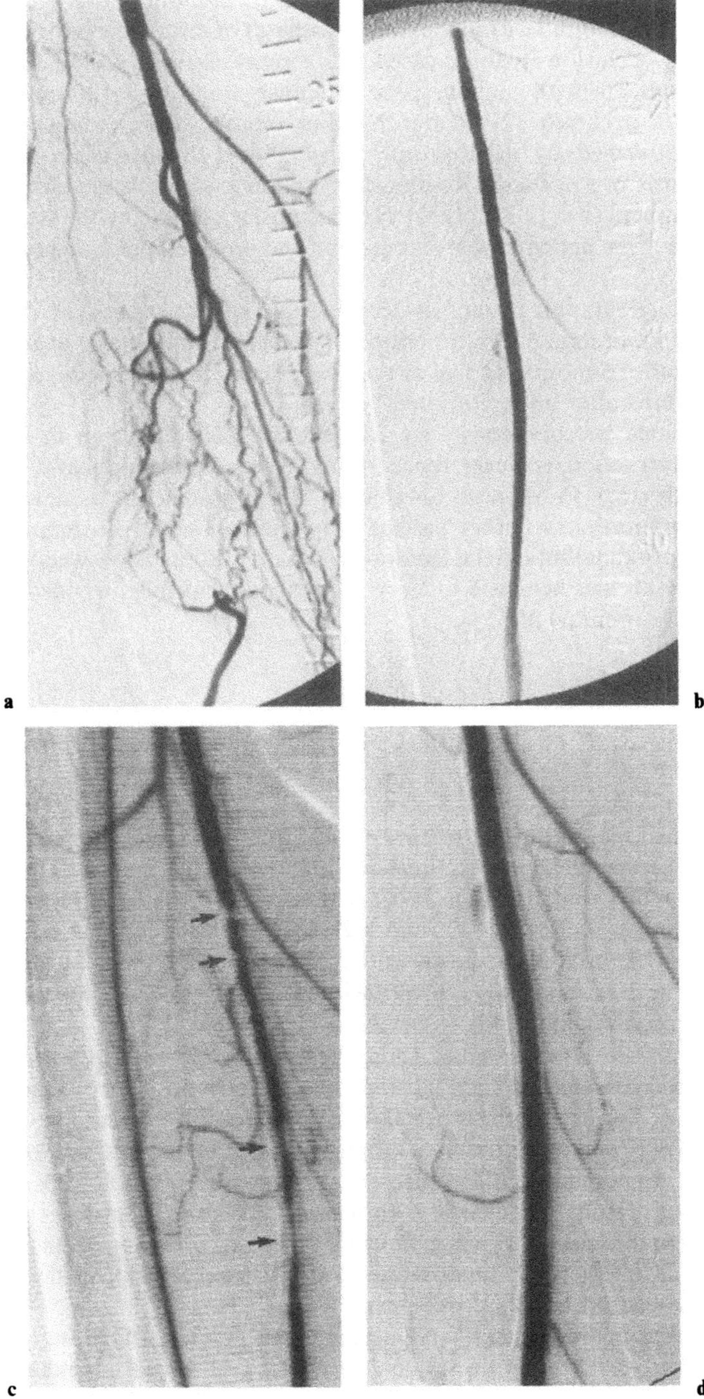

months. An overall patency rate of 94.4% was found at 12-month follow-up. Angiographic restenosis was found within the endoprostheses of seven iliac patients (6.9%) with a previous occlusion in three cases and a stenosis in four cases. In three asymptomatic patients with angiographic restenosis at 6- and 12-month intervals, late occlusion occurred 12–18 months after treatment. Percutaneous reintervention was performed by atherectomy and balloon dilatation in five patients; repeat restenosis was not seen. Restenosis within iliac stents ranged from 9–24 months after treatment ($\bar{x} = 13.3$ months). New lesions neighbouring the stent extremities occurred in three patients with iliac lesions and required percutaneous reintervention in all.

In femoral stents, angiographic restenosis occurred in 6 of 19 patients (31.5%) who were followed for more than 3 months: all patients were symptomatic again. Restenosis occurred within 6 months in five of the six patients. Restenosis did not occur later than 9 months after implantation (Fig. 5).

Restenosis was treated percutaneously by atherectomy and dilatation in all patients [21]; repeat obstruction, however, reoccurred in three of the six patients.

In one patient with stage IV disease, no change of symptoms was achieved and she underwent amputation. Another patient developed an acute thrombosis of a stent placed in the proximal superficial femoral artery after lifting heavy weights at work. A sufficient result was achieved in 11 of 20 patients, and this provided a mid-term success rate (6 months) of 55%.

4 Discussion

PTA is a well-established method in the treatment of arterial occlusive disease. It has now been widely accepted as a less invasive and expensive method than surgical treatment, but one that has high success rates [1, 2, 6, 8]. *Becker* et al. calculated a mean technical success of 92% and a 2-year patency rate of 81% for iliac PTA [1]. Even for femoral PTA, mean initial success is 89% with modern instrumentation [1]. The 2-year patency is lower, with 67%, but may be compared to results of surgical reconstruction [1].

With regard to these favourable results, it may be asked whether there is any need for a supplementary technique such as stent insertion. A positively biased selection, however, has to be assumed for lesions undergoing percutaneous treatment, because PTA is often omitted in a subset of lesions which are not well amenable to balloon angioplasty either because of early technical failure or disappointing follow-up results. Iliac artery occlusions, eccentric stenoses and orificial lesions belong to this group [1]—a group which also includes long-segment stenoses of the femoral artery [11]. The usefulness of vascular endoprostheses, therefore, has to be proved on this kind of lesion.

Results of iliac stenting have been encouraging. Although indication for endovascular prostheses was focused on lesions which are not ideally amenable to PTA alone, a high initial technical success of 98% was reached, and the 1-year patency rate exceeded 90% in our patients. Restenosis caused by intimal hyperplasia does not seem to become an important problem in iliac endoprostheses, although reobstruction tends to develop later in iliac than in femoral implants. Consequently, long-term results of 2 or 5 years will have to be taken into account before a definitive conclusion can be drawn.

Special emphasis should be put on the treatment of iliac occlusions, which have been a relatively infrequent subject in PTA until recently, because a low technical success and a considerable complication rate has been reported [14, 17]. In our opinion, self-expandable endoprostheses help to overcome technical problems with these lesions. The stent fixates the thrombotic material to the vascular wall, thus preventing it from dislodgement following PTA, and it stabilizes the vascular lumen achieved by balloon dilatation thus preventing overdilatation [24]. Contralateral and ipsilateral embolization did occur in our patients [24], but they were due to enforced dilatation following stent implantation or incomplete coverage of the occluded segment, and not to stent placement itself. We learned from that experience, however, that even with an endoprosthesis in place, overdilation has to be strictly avoided in the treatment of iliac occlusions, particularly in ostial lesions. As an alternative, combined treatment of iliac occlusions by lysis therapy and balloon dilatation may be performed. It has been reported, however, that the technical results of this procedure are no better than after mechanical revascularization, and the problem of embolization still remains [9, 16]. Moreover, this therapeutic approach is limited by general contraindications to lysis therapy [9].

Results of femoral stent placement have been disillusioning. Although a number of our patients did not show any evidence of restenosis after a long-term follow-up period, a considerable number of patients tended to develop restenosis rapidly. Repeat intervention was frequently necessary but has not yet yielded a constant success. *Triller* and co-workers [21] did not find any significant difference between femoral lesions treated with a self-expandable stent and those treated by PTA alone. Femoral stent placement generally increases costs and complicates percutaneous reintervention in case of restenosis because removal of intimal hyperplasia requires alternative and more expensive techniques than balloon angioplasty, such as atherectomy [23]. Complication rate was fairly high and was caused in particular by the thrombogenicity of the foreign body implant. Consequently, femoral stenting should be restricted to cases in which PTA obviously failed and patency of the vessel is acutely endangered by postangioplasty complications otherwise requiring bypass surgery. It seems to be unsuitable as a primary procedure in femoropopliteal arteries and is assumed to be contraindicated in areas such as the common femoral or proximal superficial femoral artery, where minor surgical intervention can be easily performed, or in vessels crossing a joint area. Restrictions might be reconsidered in case an effective supplementary medicative concept for prevention of intimal hyperplasia becomes established.

Using the self-expandable Wallstent, *Triller* et al. reported disappointing results of femoral stenting similar to ours [21]. In contrast, *Rousseau* et al. found much better results after implantation of the same type of device in the femoropopliteal arteries [18]. Mid-term results for femoral use of the Strecker stent have not yet been reported [20] and the Palmaz stent has not been routinely used in the femoral arteries, mainly for technical reasons.

For iliac stenting, a multi-center study on the Palmaz stent has been published recently reporting excellent follow-up results with this particular device [13]. With a relatively short mean follow-up time of 6 months, an overall patency of 100% was achieved. However, our own experiences have shown us that iliac reobstruction after stent implantation is more likely to appear as a late failure.

To conclude, stent placement in femoral arteries cannot be recommended as a general procedure and should be restricted to highly complex lesions or dissections which cannot be removed by other percutaneous means. The preliminary clinical experience in the iliac arteries is promising, but the importance of a reasonable cost-benefit ratio should not be neglected. Stent placement is still a costly procedure making percutaneous balloon dilatation more expensive. Consequently, stent placement should be limited to a subset of complex lesions which are not well amenable to PTA alone. Too liberal an approach to stent placement should be avoided, because it may compromise this advanced new technique by giving up the striking advantages of balloon angioplasty as a safe and successful, but also inexpensive procedure for most iliac lesions.

5 Summary

A self-expandable Wallstent was used in 123 patients as an adjunct to balloon angioplasty of complex femoral and iliac lesions. Forty-eight iliac stenoses, 55 iliac occlusions and 20 femoral lesions were treated.

The procedure showed a 98.4% success rate, with two cases of acute femoral thromboses. At 3-month follow-up two iliac lesions were reobstructed by stent thrombosis.

Further follow-up ($\bar{x} = 16.5$ months) revealed restenosis of the stented segment in seven iliac lesions (6.9%) and six femoral lesions (31.5%). Reintervention within the stents was performed combining atherectomy and balloon angioplasty in 11 cases.

Self-expandable endoprostheses proved to be a promising means of improving the technical success of complex iliac lesions. Mid-term results are encouraging but restenosis of iliac stents tends to occur beyond 6 month follow-up, thus making further follow-up studies necessary.

Stenting of femoral lesions was complicated by a high frequency of restenosis and should be carried out only on a restricted basis.

References

1. Becker GJ, Katzen BT, Dake MD (1989) Noncoronary angioplasty. Radiology 170:921–940
2. Dotter CT, Judkins MP (1964) Transluminal angioplasty of atherosclerotic obstructions: description of a new technic and a preliminary report of its application. Circulation 30:654–670
3. Dotter CT (1969) Transluminally placed coilspring endarterial tube grafts: long-term patency in canine popliteal artery. Invest Radiol 4:329–332

4. Dotter CT, Buschmann R, McKinney M, Rösch J (1983) Transluminal expandable nitinol coil stent grafting: preliminary report. Radiology 147:259–260
5. Cragg AH, Lund G, Rysavy J et al. (1984) Percutaneous arterial grafting. Radiology 150:45–49
6. Grüntzig A, Hopff M (1974) Perkutane Rekanalisation chronischer arterieller Verschlüsse mit einem neuen Dilatationskatheter: Modifikation der Dotter-Technik. Dtsch Med Wochenshr 99:2502–2510
7. Guenther RW, Vorwerk D, Bohndorf K et al. (1989) Iliac and femoral artery stenoses and occlusions: treatment with intravascular stents. Radiology 172:725–730
8. Johnston KW, Rae M, Hogg-Johnston S et al. (1987) 5-year results of a prospective study of percutaneous transluminal angioplasty. Ann Surg 206:403–410
9. Lammer J, Pilger E, Neumayer K et al. (1986) Intraarterial fibrinolysis: long-term results. Radiology 161:159–163
10. Maass D, Zollikofer CL, Largiader F, Senning A (1984) Radiological follow-up of transluminally inserted vascular endoprostheses: an experimental study using expanding spirals. Radiology 152:659–663
11. Murray RR Jr, Hewes RC, White RI Jr et al. (1987) Long-segment femoropopliteal stenoses: is angioplasty a boon or a bust? Radiology 162:473–478
12. Palmaz JC, Sibbitt R, Reuter S et al. (1985) Expandable intraluminal graft: a preliminary study. Radiology 156:73–77
13. Palmaz JC, Garcia O, Schatz R et al. (1990) Placement of balloon-expandable intraluminal stents in iliac arteries: first 171 procedures. Radiology 174:969–975
14. Pilla T, Peterson G, Tantana S, Lang E et al (1984) Percutaneous recanalization of iliac artery occlusions: an alternative to surgery in the high-risk patient. AJR 143:313–316
15. Rabkin J (1989) Roentgenendoprosthetics of the vessels, biliary ducts, bronchus, trachea and uterus with nitinol prosthesis. 6th Grazer Symposium, 12.-14.10.89, Grz
16. Rees CR, Palmaz JC, Garcia O et al (1989) Angioplasty and stenting of completely occluded iliac arteries. Radiology 172:953–959
17. Ring E, Freiman D, McLean G, Schwarz W (1982) Percutaneous recanalization of iliac artery occlusions: an unacceptable complication rate. AJR 39:587–589
18. Rousseau H, Raillat C, Joffre F et al. (1989) Treatment of femoropopliteal stenoses by means of self-expandable endoprostheses: midterm results. Radiology 172:961–964
19. Sigwart U, Puel J, Mirkovitch V et al. (1987) Intravascular stents to prevent occlusion and restenosis after transluminal angioplasty. N Engl J Med 316:701–706
20. Strecker E, Romaniuk R, Schneider B et al. (1988) Perkutan implantierbare, durch Ballon aufdehnbare Gefäss prothese. Dtsch Med Wochenschr 113:538–542
21. Triller J, Mahler F, Do D, Thalmann R (1989) Die vaskulaere Endoprothese bei femoropoplitealer Verschlusskrankheit. Fortschr Roentgenstr 150:328–334
22. Wright KC, Wallace S, Charnsangavej C et al. (1985) Percutaneous endovascular stent: an experimental evaluation. Radiology 156:69–72
23. Vorwerk D, Guenther RW (1990) Removal of intimal hyperplasia in vascular endoprostheses managed by combined use of atherectomy and balloon dilatation. AJR 154:617–619
24. Vorwerk D, Guenther RW (1990) Mechanical revascularization of occluded iliac arteries with use of self-expandable endoprostheses. Radiology 175:411–415

Laser-Induced Shock Wave Angioplasty: Discrimination Between Calcified and Other Plaque Material Before Generation of Laser-Induced Shock Waves

M. Zwaan[1], M. Scheu[2], A. Lebeau[1], J.H. Göthlin[3], R. Engelhardt[2], and H.-D. Weiss[1]

1 Introduction

Percutaneous dilatation of stenotic vessels was first reported by *Dotter* [1] in 1964. *Grüntzig's* [2] balloon angioplasty is employed daily in interventional radiological centers. The results in complete obstructions longer than 5 cm are discouraging. The results are negatively correlated with length, degree of calcification, and duration of the occlusion.

Laser angioplasty has been attempted for recanalization of arteriosclerotic arteries by destroying plaques with laser radiation, transmitted through light guides [3]. Argon [4–6] and excimer laser systems [7–10] are already established, while pulsed dye [11–17], holmium [18], and alexandrite lasers [17] are now being tested.

Calcified plaques can be disintegrated by photoablation (e.g., excimer laser) or shock waves generated by laser-induced plasma (e.g., pulsed dye or alexandrite laser). Both methods carry high risk of perforation caused by the inability to precisely target the laser energy to the diseased parts of the vessel only [3, 19, 22].

[1] Departments of Radiology and Pathology, Medical University of Lübeck, Ratzeburger Allee 160, W-2400 Lübeck, Germany
[2] Medical Laser Center Lübeck, Peter-Monnik-Weg 9, W-2400 Lübeck, Germany
[3] Department of Radiology, University of Göteborg, Sahlgrenska Hospital, S-41345 Göteborg, Sweden

Frontiers in European Radiology, Vol. 8
Eds. Baert/Heuck
© Springer-Verlag, Berlin Heidelberg 1991

Several attempts have been made to overcome this by spectroscopic means, e.g., analysis of the plasma flash or laser-induced fluorescence (LIF) [23–26].

In order to study the discrimination between normal intima and calcified lesions by the intensity of LIF signals, we used a pulsed dye laser at 495 nm.

2 Materials and Methods

2.1 Arterial Tissue Samples

In total, 376 artery samples were excised from fresh human cadavers and frozen. Investigation was performed with normal intima (group A), fibro-fatty plaques (group B), white calcified plaques (group C), and hemorrhagic ulcerated lesions (group D). Histologic examination of specimens was performed and radiograms obtained to discriminate calcified from noncalcified parts. In the first 50 specimens histology examination was performed, but as the results were well correlated with the radiograms and visual inspection, no further histology was obtained.

2.2 LIF Spectroscopy

A pulsed dye laser operated at 495 nm, pulse length 1 μs, was used. Figure 1 demonstrates the experimental setup. The laser emission was transmitted through an optical fiber with a diameter of 250 μm, the tip of which was in direct contact with the samples. The same fiber was used to emit and receive fluorescence signal. The fluorescent light was transformed into an electrical signal by a photodiode with a bypass filter (OG 515) in front of the photodiode. The photodiode signal was then displayed on a fast-strorage oscilloscope, triggered by the laser pulse itself allowing a spectral integration. All measurements were performed in air. The

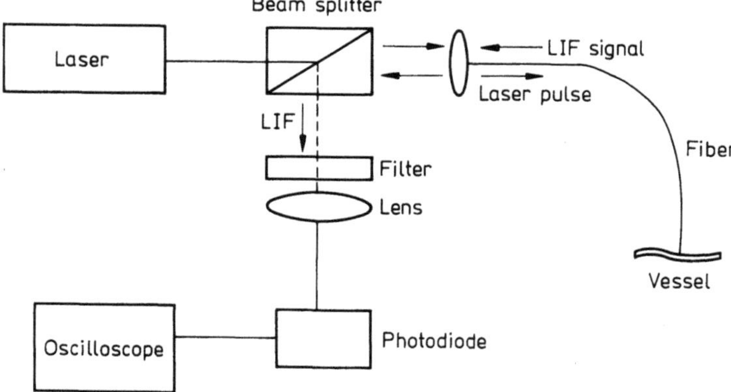

Fig. 1. Experimental setup to detect the LIF signal

laser energy was kept constant. The relative fluorescence of the different specimens were compared at 250 ns after onset of laser pulse.

2.3 Particle Sizing

To assess the possible complication of particle embolization we measured the size of particles resulting from the shock wave procedure. Three samples of each group (A, B, C, and D) were subjected to 500 shock waves at 495 nm, with energies of either 30, 50 or 60 mJ, respectively.

The particles were washed out with physiological saline, centrifuged at 2000 rpm over 2 min and counted in a hemocytometer. The particles were also investigated microscopically and photographed to assess particle size (Olympus objective micrometer).

2.4 Tissue Effects

The laser plasma ablation created at 50 mJ, 495 nm, was histologically investigated.

2.5 Laser Recanalization

Angiography of five excised human arteries was performed to document obstruction. The laser fiber was inserted through a flexible catheter with a blunt tip. When resistance was encountered, shock waves were induced and the catheter, with laser fiber, thereafter advanced until no obstruction was felt. The recanalization was documented angiographically.

3 Results

3.1 Fluorescence Intensity of Tissue Samples

Figure 2 shows the relative fluorescence intensities of the different groups A, B, C, and D for excitation at 495 nm. The vertical (intensity) scale is plotted in arbitrary units, as the absolute scale depends on several experimental parameters such as laser energy, filter transmission, and sensitivity of the photodiode. But for our analysis the detection of the relative intensity differences between progressive stages of vascular disease is the parameter of interest.

There is an obvious discrimination level between healthy intima (A), fibro-fatty plaques (B), and ulcerated plaques (D) on one side and calcified lesions (C) on the other. It is possible to select a discrimination level in such a way that none of the group A, B, and D specimens will be detected as calcified in a feedback system based on LIF intensity. When applying this discrimination level there were no false-positive signals in groups A and B (A × 0/30; B × 0/30), respectively. In group C the discrimination level could not be reached in two samples (2/20). In group

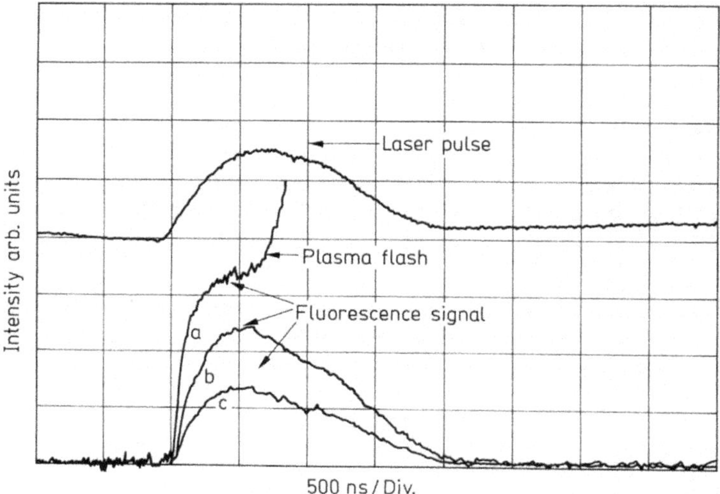

Fig. 2. Different fluorescence signals. In (*a*) the resulting signal of calcified plaque material is higher than healthy intima (*b*) and fibro-fatty plaques (*c*). Before plasma ignition a fluorescence signal is detected, *X-axis*, intensity in arbitrary (arb.) units; *y-axis*, 500 ns per division (div.)

D there were 18 discrimination-level crossings in 286 samples. These 18 specimens reacted like calcified plaques and were shown to contain calcifications.

3.2 Particle Sizing

At each energy level the shock wave-created particles were more than 99% smaller than $10\,\mu$m. However, some fragments were about 1 mm and in group A consisted of shreds of tissue and in the other groups, in addition, calcium and cholesterol crystals.

The microparticles in group A contained whole and fragmented endothelium cells and erythrocytes. In group B, additionally, were observed cholesterin crystals and parts of them (Fig. 3). In groups C and D the microscopic image changed to a predominance of calcium crystals (Fig. 4).

3.3 Tissue Effects

The laser energies employed produced sharply demarcated lesions with a maximum depth of about a quarter of the intima thickness (Fig. 5). There was no carbonization, but a minimal coagulation adjacent to the laser crater walls.

3.4 Laser Recanalization

Five totally occluded arteries (proved at arteriography) were recanalized with a bare fiber (Fig. 6). The shock wave impulse softened the obstruction and thus made a subsequent mechanical recanalization possible.

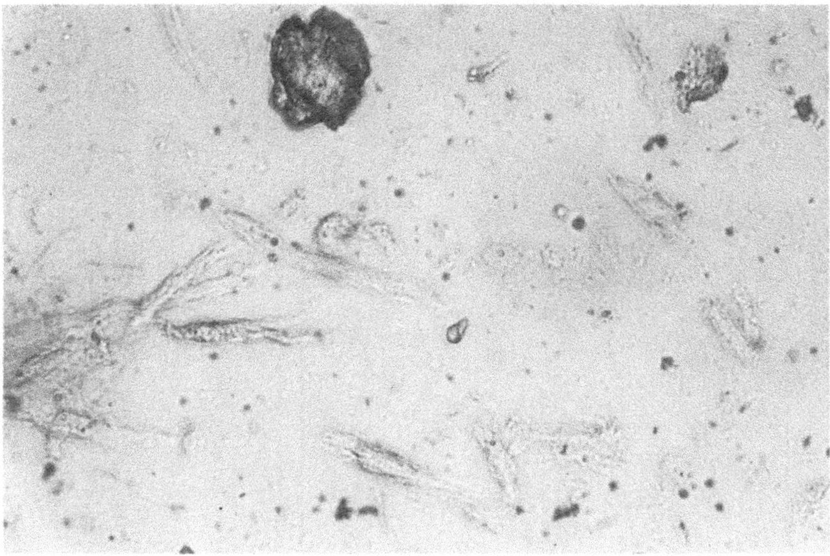

Fig. 3. Centrifuged cholesterol crystals created by laser-induced shock waves to fibro-fatty plaque material

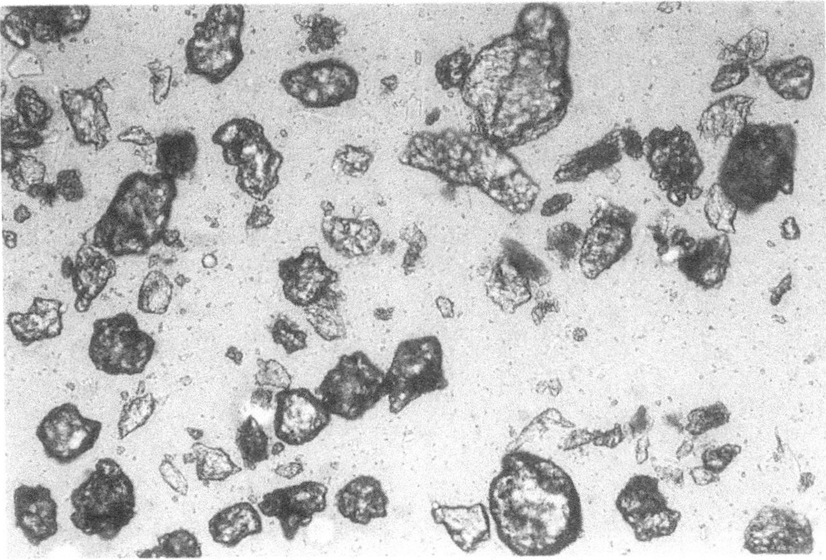

Fig. 4. Centrifuged calcium crystals created by laser-induced shock waves to calcified plaques and hemorrhagic ulcerated lesions

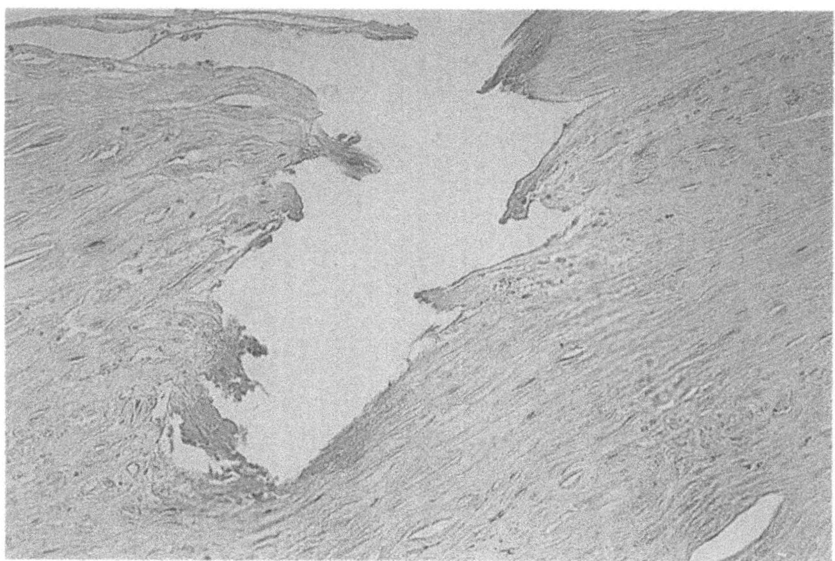

Fig. 5. Tissue defect after laser ablation with a dye laser at 50 mJ. There is no carbonization, but a minimal coagulation at the laser crater walls

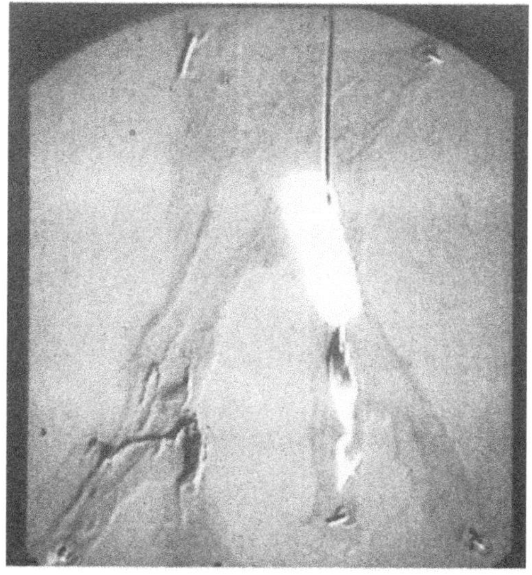

Fig. 6. Angiography of a recanalized totally occluded internal iliac artery with a bare fiber in an experimental setup

4 Discussion

The investigation shows that at least in vitro the intensity of the LIF signal can be used to discriminate calcified lesions from normal arterial tissue at an excitation wave length of 495 nm. Furthermore, using time-resolved detection of the fluorescent light, the laser power can be switched off at the beginning of the laser pulse when noncalcified artery tissue is detected in front of the fiber. Thus, detection and disintegration of plaques can be performed with the same laser fiber. If the system failed, only a minimal intima destruction would be expected (M.R. Prince, personal communication).

We have found that a path can be created through long artery occlusions without having to first pass a guide wire. When the occlusion has been opened, a guide wire and mechanical devices can be used for conventional dilatation. It is not unlikely that in the near future lasers will be used to create channels in totally obstructed arteries to permit subsequent mechanical recanalization.

The embolization risk is a real problem. We are attempting to create a rinsing/suction catheter system to overcome this problem.

Conclusively, it may be said that pulsed radiation from a dye laser at 495 nm in vitro has minimal effects on healthy artery walls at 50 mJ, even without a self-limiting system, but that totally occluded arteries may be opened for subsequent mechanical dilatation. However, as shown in other studies, bare fibers may carry a considerable perforation risk.

5 Summary

A pulsed dye laser operated at 495 nm was employed to study discrimination between normal intima and calcified artery wall lesions by the intensity of laser-induced fluorescence (LIF) signals. The material consisted of 376 aorta and artery wall cadaver specimens, which included normal intima, fibro-fatty plaques, white calcified plaques, and ulcerated lesions. At excitation with 495 nm a significant intensity discrimination level in the LIF intensity was demonstrated. A correct classification of calcified plaques and normal intima wall was obtained in vitro.

Particle sizing studies showed that more than 99% of shock wave—destroyed calcified plaque fragments were smaller than 10 μm. The few fragments with a size about 1 mm or larger may constitute an embolization risk.

In vitro investigation of explanted totally occluded human arteries showed that recanalization without the use of guide wire is possible.

LIF with a pulsed dye laser system may also, in vivo, recanalize totally occluded arteriosclerotic vessels without guide wire and with small risk of perforation.

References

1. Dotter CT, Judkins MP (1964) Transluminal treatment of atherosclerotic obstructions: description of a new technique and a preliminary report of its application. Circulation 30:654–670
2. Grüntzig A (1974) Perkutane Rekanalization chronischer arterieller Verschlüsse mit einem neuen Dilatations-Katheter. Modifikation der Dotter-Technik. Dtsch Med Wochenschr 99:2502
3. Ginsburg R, Wexler L, Mitchell RS, Profitt D (1985) Percutaneous transluminal laser angioplasty for treatment of peripheral vascular disease. Radiology 156:619–624
4. Abela GS, Seeger JM, Barbieri E, Franzini D, Fenech A, Pepine CJ, Conti CR (1986) Laser angioplasty with angioscopic guidance in humans. J Am Coll Cardiol 8:184–192
5. Choy DSJ, Sterzer SH, Myler RK, Marco J, Fournial G (1984) Human coronary laser recanalization. Clin Cardiol 7:377–381
6. Matsumoto T, Naide D, Schafer C, Harad AS, DuPree J, Yang Y (1988) Laser angioplasty. Surg Gynecol Obstet 166:81–83
7. Huppert PE, Duda SH, Haase KK, Karsch KR, Claussen CD (1990) Eximer-Laser-Angioplastie. ROFO 152:259–263
8. Karsch KR, Mauser M, Voelker W, Haase KK, Ickrath O, Duda S, Seipel L (1989) Percutaneous coronary excimer laser angioplasty. Initial clinical results. Lancet ii:647–650
9. Lammer J, Pilger E, Kleinert R, Ascher PW (1987) Laser-Angioplastie peripherer arterieller Verschlüsse. ROFO 147:119–123
10. Litvak F, Grundfest WS, Goldenberg T, Laudenslager J, Forrester JJ (1989) Percutaneous excimer laser angioplasty of aortocoronary saphenous vein grafts. J Am Coll Cardiol 14:803–808
11. Leon MB, LU DY, Prevosti LG, Macy WW, Smith PD, Granovsky M, Bonner RF, Balaban RS (1988) Human arterial surface flourescence: atherosclerotic plaque identification and effects of laser atheroma ablation. J Am Coll Cardiol 12:94–102
12. Murray A, Crocker PR, Wood RFM (1988) The pulsed dye laser and atherosclerotic vascular disease. Br J Surg 75:349–351
13. Murray A, Basu R, Wells C, Wood RMF (1989) Defining parameters for peripheral laser angioplasty. Eur J Vasc Surg 3:31–36
14. Murray A, Mitchell DC, Grasty M, Wood RMF, Edwards DH, Basu R (1989) Peripheral laser angioplasty with pulsed dye laser and ball-tipped optical fibres. Lancet ii:1471–1474
15. Prince MR, Deutsch TF, Mathews-Roth MM, Margolis R, Parrish JA, Oseroff AR (1986) Preferential light absorption in atheromas in vitro. J Clin Invest 78:295–302
16. Prince MR, Muraglia GM, MacNichol EFjr (1988) Increased preferential absorption in human atherosclerotic plaque with oral beta carotene. Implications for laser endarterectomy. Circulation 78:338–344
17. Scheu M, Engelhardt R, Göthlin HJ (1990) Detection of calcified plaques before generation of laser-induced shockwaves: dye laser, alexandrite laser. SPIE Optical Fibers in Medicine V 1201:38–45
18. Lilge L, Radtke W, Nishioka NS (1989) Pulsed holmium laser ablation of cardiac valves. Lasers Surg Med 9:458–464
19. Grundfest WS, Litvack F, Sherman T, Carroll R, Lee M, Chaux A, Kass R, Matloff J, Berci G, Swan HJC, Morgenstern L, Forrester J (1985) Delineation of peripheral and coronary detail by intraoperative angioscopy. Ann Surg 202 (suppl 3):394–400
20. Abela GS, Fenech A, Crea F, Conti CR (1985) "Hot tip": another method of laser vascular recanalization. Lasers Surg Med 5:327–335
21. Motarjeme A (1987) Percutaneous laser angioplasty: update after 1 year. Radiology 165 (p):240
22. Nordstrom LA, Castaneda-Zuniga WR, Young EG, von Seggern KB (1988) Direct argon laser exposure for recanalization of peripheral arteries: early results. Radiology 168:359–364
23. Bhatta KM, Rosen DI, Dretler SP (1989) Acoustic and plasma-guided laser angioplasty. Laser Surg Med 9:117–123
24. Deckelbaum LI, Lam JK, Cabin HS, Clubb KS, Long MB (1987) Discrimination of normal and atherosclerotic aorta by laser-induced fluorescence. Laser Surg Med 7:330–335
25. Deckelbaum LI, Stetz ML, O'Brien KM, Cutruzzola FW, Gmitro AF, Laifer LI, Gindi GR (1989) Fluorescence spectroscopy guidance of laser ablation of atherosclerotic plaque. Laser Surg Med 9:205–214
26. Laufer G, Wollenek G, Hohla K, Horvat R, Henke K-H, Buchelt M, Wutzl G, Wolner E (1988) Excimer laser-induced simultaneous ablation and spectral identification of normal and atherosclerotic arterial tissue layers. Circulation 78:1031–1039

Contrast Agents in Clinical Angiography—Relevance to Thromboembolic Phenomena

P. Dawson

1 Introduction

Accidental embolisation of the patient is one of the clinical angiographer's greatest fears, particularly in the coronary and cerebral territories where the result may be, naturally, disastrous. Emboli may be composed of air, talc from gloves [1], fibres from swabs [1–3], particulate contaminants always found in contrast agents and flushing solutions [1], cholesterol [4, 5], and clots that have formed during the procedure either in or on catheter/syringe/guideline systems. This last form of embolism, which has been discussed most in the literature [6–11], is the one which can, in principle, be most easily minimised by good technique [8, 12, 13]. The specific phenomenon of thromboembolism, and the factors which may contribute to it, have also formed the basis of great controversy recently, particularly in the United States, as it has been suggested that there is a greater risk associated with the in all other ways better and safer non-ionic contrast agents [13, 14].

In this article the background to these matters will be discussed and the interactions between iodinated intravascular contrast agents and blood will be reviewed in order to clarify the status of non-ionic contrast agents in clinical angiography.

2 Thromboembolic Phenonema

Thromboembolism in angiography is not a new phenomenon but has long been a recognised and, to some extent, a well-understood and feared phenomenon. Not surprisingly, most studies have been made in the context of cerebral (and coronary)

Department of Radiology, Hammersmith Hospital, Du Cone Road, London W 12 ONN, UK

Frontiers in European Radiology, Vol. 8
Eds. Baert/Heuck
© Springer-Verlag, Berlin Heidelberg 1991

angiography; thromboembolism is estimated to be responsible for the approx. 0.2% cases of distal embolisation in the leg when femoral arteriography is performed, the approx. 0.4% cases of cerebral embolisation in cerebral angiography, and the approx. 0.25% embolic events in coronary angiography. The most detailed studies have been made in coronary angiography. In the 1970s *Adams* et al. [8] noted a greater incidence of both myocardial infarct and cerebral embolisation during coronary angiography performed using the transfemoral as opposed to the transbrachial route; the respective figures using the brachial approach were 0.22% and 0.03%, while there was an incidence of 1.01% and 0.43% respectively when the femoral approach was used. Similar figures were produced in other series by a number of authors [7,9–11], and all indicated that thromboembolic events contributed significantly to morbidity and mortality in coronary angiography.

Judkins and *Gander* [12] examined all available data from a number of series and suggested that the femoral approach was apparently preferred to the brachial approach by less skilled personnel and was not ordinarily performed with systemic heparinization. The brachial approach, on the other hand, usually entailed systemic heparinization because of the well-recognised danger of the procedure to the brachial artery. It was further noted that the incidence of supposed thromboembolic complications could be up to ten times higher in centres performing relatively few examinations than in those performing larger numbers. *Judkins* and *Gander* stressed the need to reduce procedure time, to use skilled personnel or, at least, provide good supervision of less experienced personnel, to use less thrombogenic meterials as far as was possible, and to use systemic heparinization. Since the use of heparin is not without controversy, even today [15], it is important to emphasise that *Judkins* and *Gander* stressed most of all that technique and experience were the most important factors in avoiding these disasters.

At the end of the 1970s, *Adams* and *Abrams* [16] reviewed a large number of patients undergoing coronary arteriography and noted a marked reduction in the number of fatal complications usually associated with the femoral approach to a level close to that found with the brachial approach. The authors ascribed this partly to a more widespread use of systemic heparinization and partly to a greater expertise on the part of operators. This, and a number of other series at about the same time [17–19], led to a general acceptance that the incidence of thromboembolic complications in coronary angiography might be approximately 0.25% in good hands and should not be significantly greater but that the incidence could, in less experienced hands, be up to ten times higher.

It was felt at at this time, and is widely believed today, that systemic heparinization of patients may play some role in reducing thromboembolic complications but hard evidence is lacking. Even today, the use of systemic heparinization has not been rationalized and, when it is used, there is no consensus on dosage regimes. It is, in any case, now known that the heparin "requirement" of different patients varies widely [15].

In the 1970s, an interest was also shown in the role of catheters and guidewires in the aetiology of thromboembolic events [20–28]. Many studies indicated that the formation of thrombus depended on the catheter material and area (size/gauge); their occurrence was greatest where Teflon-coated materials were used and least in the case of polyethylene materials, with polyurethane materials occupying the middle position. It should be noted though that even when different manufacturers use the same material the result is not always the same, in that the surface morphology and irregularity play an important role. Heparin-impregnated catheters appear to have demonstrable advantages, but are very expensive [24, 27].

It should be noted that at this time, as evidenced by the literative, intravascular contrast agents were perceived as part of the solution and not as part of the problem. They were recognised widely by angiographers as essentially anti-coagulant materials and, indeed, it was recommended by some authors that they should be used as flushing solutions during angiography [29].

3 Newer Contrast Materials

The 1980s saw the introduction into clinical practice, first in Europe and later in the United States, of the new generation of intravascular iodinated contrast agents. These could be divided into two chemical types: the second generation non-ionic monomeric agents [the first-generation agent was metrizamide (Amipaque)], and a monoacid dimeric agent ioxaglate [30]. These were all low osmolality agents with a lower toxicity than the conventional higher osmolality agents which preceded them but it was soon established that ioxaglate was of somewhat higher toxicity than the non-ionics. However, this was only clearly expressed clinically when it was used intravenously. As an arteriographic agent is seemed to be, broadly speaking, as acceptable as the non-ionic agents and, indeed, in some cases where arteriography was painful, generally better in view of its slightly lower osmolality.

In both Europe and the United States, the non-ionic agents became more firmly established generally speaking, than ioxaglate and evidence began to emerge that the non-ionics specifically were safer in terms of being associated with a reduced incidence of major anaphylactoid reactions—at least on intravenous injection. Probably the only factor which prevented their general use in most countries was their high price.

This relatively simple situation became complicated for the angiographer in 1987 when two intriguing reports appeared, one in the Scandinavian literature [31] and one in the American literature [13]. The first paper by *Raininko* [31] explained that non-ionic contrast agents in contact with blood could engender a disordered red cell aggregation phenomenon rather akin to that seen with dextrose solutions in contact with blood [32]. Although the observation was made in vitro it was argued that if such aggregates forming in catheters and syringes were to be reinjected into the patient, or were formed in vivo, then accidental embolisation of the patient might be a danger. The second paper by *Robertson* [13] suggested that when blood contaminates a contrast-containing syringe, a clot is more likely to form if the contrast agent concerned is a non-ionic agent. The risk of such a clot formating, with consequent reinjection and accidental embolisation of the patient, it was said, would therefore be greater with the non-ionic agents. These reports, particularly the latter, caused the the greatest controversy in American radiology for half a century. Interestingly, though, very little interest was generated in Europe. The explanation for this may lie, at least partly, in the special medico-legal climate in which American angiographers must work. It must also be said that, for the most part, more heat than light was generated in this controversy, but it did have the positive effect of stimulating angiographers to think about their technique and to re-examine previous knowledge concerning blood-contrast agent interactions. It also encouraged some genuinely new studies which produced interesting and useful information.

We can summarise our present knowledge about contrast agent and blood interactions, in so far as it bears on the question of thromboembolism, as follows:

1. All iodinated contrast media, old and new, are essentially anticoagulant. They inhibit the coagulation cascade at a number of levels, in particular but not exclusively, by inhibiting fibrin polymerisation.
2. All intravascular contrast agents inhibit the aggregation of platelets.
3. Nothing was known prior to 1987, and no evidence has emerged since, to indicate that there is any qualitative difference in the effects of different kinds of contrast agents on blood. The differences are quantitative, the non-ionic agents having less effect on the coagulation cascade and platelet aggregation, entirely as might be predicted because of their greater biocompatibility [33].
4. Absolutely no evidence has emerged to suggest any "pro-coagulant" or "pro-thrombotic" effects from non-ionic (or other) contrast agents. Notwithstanding this last fact, a number of recent contributions to the literature have, unfortunately, made use of such terms with absolutely no foundation in any data and in a manner likely to generate anxiety among angiographers.
5. The lower effect of the non-ionic agents on the coagulation cascade and platelet aggregation does appear to lead, as would be expected, to a somewhat increased likelihood of thrombus formation in catheters and syringes than is the case when ionic agents, old or new, are used. However, it is important to retain the right perspective in all this. First of all when *Dawson* et al. [34] attempted to reproduce *Robertson's* results by contaminating various contrast containing syringes with blood, it was found very difficult to produce clots in any contrast agent. It would appear that some effort and an exceptionally bad technique has to be used to generate such clots. Furthermore, it is equally important to realise that there was no indication, let alone data, from actual clinical angiography of there being any problem with the non-ionics. They had been used since the beginning of the 1980s in Europe, in some countries almost exclusively, and in the United States from 1985. Indeed, adverse reaction reports made to the Food and Drug Administration in the 2 years or so following *Robertson's* article indicated that there was actually a higher incidence of thromboembolic phenomena associated with the ionic agent, ioxaglate, than with the non-ionics! [14]. This should, of course, be viewed with great caution as such reporting systems are, it is well known, not at all perfect, and at a time of anxiety and confusion over a new group of drugs a fair degree of inaccurate and confused reporting is only to be expected.

Some new information did emerge from studies stimulated by this controversy. *Dawson* et al. [34, 35] reported that, not surprisingly, glass syringes are highly thrombogenic and, where possible, are best avoided in clinical angiography, but also indicated that not all plastics are the same. Strene acrylonitrile is, for example, more thrombogenic than its counter part polypropylene.

Although a good deal of work has been done in the past on catheter materials, little has been done recently and, given that there have been a number of changes in materials and construction in recent years, some new studies would appear to be in order.

4 Technique

If the problem of clots forming in syringes is to be prevented, it is obvious that the contamination of syringes with blood should be avoided as far as possible. This is, however, a counsel of perfection; contamination will occur and when it does, the syringe and its contents should not be left for any length of time before injection and should, in any case, be inspected briefly for any obvious clot before use. As far as catheters are concerned, as rapid a procedure as is reasonably possible must be performed in order to minimise the extent to which a clot may form on the outer surface of the catheter, and frequent flushing must be performed to prevent the buildup of a clot on its inner surface. In the latter regard, frequent and vigorous intermittent flushing is more important than considerations of whether or not the flushing solution is heparinized and by how much. Indeed, there may be some danger in the elaborate continuous heparinized flush systems used by some angiographers and cardiologists as they may lull the operator into a false sense of security. This particularly applies in the case of multiple side-hole catheters which, when the flush pressure is insufficient, may only have their side-holes (or sometimes only the proximal side-holes in multiple side-hole systems) flushed rather than the end-hole. A thrombus may consequently build up at the tip. This is especially true of pigtail catheters and such a thrombus forming in the end may well be dislodged by the first really vigorous injection of contrast by hand or pump.

5 Summary

Whatever precautions are taken and whatever technique, materials, and contrast agents are used, thromboembolic phenomena will occasionally occur and will sometimes be disastrous. The incidence should be less than 0.25% and in any centre where it is not, procedural considerations should be re-examined. The role of contrast agents of any kind, as far as is known, is a helpful one in this regard since all contrast agents, including the non-ionics, are anticoagulant. The non-ionics are, indeed, less anticoagulant than are the ionics and, therefore, there is little doubt that the likelihood of clot formation in catheters and syringes containing these agents is somewhat greater than in those containing the ionics; the increased risk, however, appears to be small and does not appear to have manifested itself in any obvious way in actual clinical angiography. Some of the recent literature in this field is not only confusing but positively misleading.

On the subject of catheter materials, we may say that the thrombogenicity of some of the newer catheter materials warrants investigation and more thought should be given to the development of better catheter materials and to surface morphology by the companies involved.

In the case of angioplasty it may be best to reserve judgement on the relative merits of different contrast agents. No data are available but it seems reasonable to hypothesise that the special environment created in angioplasty as a result of a grossly injured endothelium and periods of relative and absolute stasis—sometimes for prolonged periods—may warrant the use of both systemic heparinization and the most anticoagulant contrast agents available.

As for systemic heparinization, there is general feeling that it is helpful but that large-scale trials are needed to establish this. Even if heparinization were proven to be useful it would be necessary to establish meaningful methods of controlling its effectiveness during procedures—determining activated whole blood clotting time, for example.

Non-ionic contrast agents are better tolerated than their ionic counterparts and are, on the basis of first principles, to be preferred in general. They are costly and therefore some discrimination in their use is not unreasonable, but to deprive those patients who would benefit from them because of some poorly founded concern that they are somehow pro-coagulant would seem unjustified.

Perhaps we can do no better than to quote *Bettmann* [36]: "experience suggests that these differences in clotting (between ionics and non-ionics) are far less important than the combination of training, judgement and careful adherence to optimal technique".

The key to safe angiography is good technique, not bad contrast agents.

References

1. Winding O (1987) Contaminants in contrast media and catheters. In: Ansell G, Wilkins RA (eds) Complications in diagnostic imaging, 2nd edn. Blackwell, Oxford, pp 430–439
2. Adams DF, Olin TB, Kose KJ (1965) Cotton fibre embolisation during angiography. Radiology 165:678–681
3. Kay JM, Wilkins RA (1969) Cotton fibre embolisation during angiography. Clin Radiol 20:410–413
4. Ramirez G, O'Neill WM, Lambert R, Bloom MA (1978) Cholesterol embolisation: a complication of angiography. Arch Int Med 138:1430–1432
5. Perdue GD, Smith RB (1969) Atheromatous microemboli. Ann Surgery 169:954–959
6. Formanek G, Frech RS, Amplatz K (1970) Arterial thrombus formation during clinical percutaneous catheterisation. Circulation 41:833–839
7. Green GS, McKinnon CM, Roech j (1972) Complications of selective percutaneous coronary arteriography and their prevention. A review of 445 consecutive examinations. Circulation 45:552–557
8. Adams DF, Fraser DB, Abrams HC (1973) The complication of coronary arteriography. Circulation 48:609–612
9. Takaro T, Pifarre R, Wuerflein RD (1972) Acute coronary occlusion following coronary arteriography. Mechanism and surgical relief. Surgery 72:1018–1029
10. Takaro T, Hultgren HH, Littman D (1973) An analysis of deaths occurring in association with coronary arteriography. Am Heart J 86:587–597

11. De la Torre, Jacobs D, Aleman J Anderson GA (1973) Embolic coronary artery occlusion in percutaneous transfemoral coronnary arteriography. Am Heart J 86:467473
12. Judkins MP, Gander MP (1974) Complications of coronary arteriography. Circulation 49:599–602
13. Robertson HJF (1987) Blood clot formation in angiographic syringes containing non-ionic contrast media. Radiology 162:621–622
14. Robertson HJF (1988) Non-ionic contrast media in radiology. Procedural considerations. Invest Radiol 23:S374–S377
15. Miller DL (1989) Heparin in angiography: current patterns of use. Radiology 172:1007–1011
16. Adams DF, Abrams HL (1979) Complications of coronary arteriography: a follow-up report. Cardiovasc Radiol 2:89–92
17. Davis K, Kennedy JW, Kemp MG, Judkins MP (1979) Complications of coronary arteriography from the collaborative study of coronary artery surgery (CASS). Circulation 59:1105–1112
18. Kennedy JW (1982) Mortality related to cardiac catheterisation and angiography. Cathet Cardiovasc Diagn 8:323–327
19. Kennedy JW (1982) Complications associated with cardiac catheterisation and angiography. Cathet Cardiovasc Diagn 8:5–9
20. Björk L (1972) Heparin coating of catheter against thromboembolism in percutaneous catheterisation for angiography. Acta Radiol [Diagn] 12:576–578
21. McCarty RJ, Glasser SP (1973) Thrombogenicity of guidewires. Am J Cardiol 32:943–946
22. Duitt TW, Durst S, Moore R, Amplatz K (1974) Guidewire thrombogenicity and its reduction. Radiology 111:43–46
23. Durst S, Johnson BS, Amplatz K (1974) The effect of silicone coatings on thrombogenicity. Am J Reontgenol 120:904–906
24. Eldh P, Jacobsson B (1974) Heparinised vascular catheters. A clinical trial. Radiology 111:289–292
25. Bourassa MG, Cantin M, Sandborn EB, Pederson E (1976) Scanning electron microscopy of surface irregularities and thrombogenesis of polyurethane andpolyethylene coronary catheters. Circulation 53:992–996
26. Wilner GD, Casarella WJ, Baier R (1978) Thrombogenicity of angiographic catheters. Circ Res 43:424–429
27. Kido DK, Paulin S, Aienghat JA, Wafernaux C, Riley LD (1982) Thrombogenicity of heparin and non-heparin coated catheter: clinical trial. Am J Roentgenol 139:957–961
28. Judkins MP, Hinck VC, Dotter CT (1968) Teflon-coated safety guides. An adjunct to the use of polyurethane catheters. Am J Roentgenol 104:223–224
29. Hawkins IF, Herbert L (1974) Contrast material used as catheter flushing agent: a method to reduce clot formation during angiography. Radiology 110:351–352
30. Dawson P, Pitfield J, Grainger RG (1983) The low osmolality contrast agents. A simple guide. Clin Radiol 34:221–226
31. Raininko R, Ylinen SL (1987) Effect of ionic and non-ionic contrast media on aggregation of red blood cells in vitro. Acta Radiol [Diagn] 28:87–92
32. Wilson H (1950) Aqueous dextrose solutions. A hazard in transfusion. Am J Clin Pathol 20:667–669
33. Dawson P (1985) Chemotoxicity of contrast agents and clinical adverse effects. Invest Radiol 20:584–591
34. Dawson P (1988) Non-ionic contrast agents and coagulation. Invest Radiol 23:S310–S317
35. Dawson P, McCarthy P, Allison DJ, Bradshaw A, Garvey B (1988) Non-ionic contrast agents, red cell aggregation and coagulation. Br J Radiol 61:963–965
36. Bettman MA (1989) Guidelines for use of low osmolality contrast agents. Radiology 172:901–903

Sodium and Oxygen Addition to Nonionic Contrast Media. Effects on Contractile Force and Risk of Ventricular Fibrillation in the Isolated Rabbit Heart

L. Bååth

1 Introduction

When investigating patients with myocardial ischemia and arteriosclerotic changes in the coronary arteries, cardioangiography and coronary angiography are of great importance. As cardiac bypass operations increase in number, so the number of these preoperative investigations is also increasing [35]. Older and more severely diseased patients than those studied previously are being investigated, for instance in connection with myocardial infarction [15]. With more vulnerable patients, it is important that the already low risks of coronary angiography become even lower and that the contrast medium used has as small a negative effect as possible.

In cardioangiography the contrast medium solution is injected into the heart chambers or the aortic bulb and a mixture of contrast medium and blood will flow through the coronary arteries. In selective coronary angiography the contrast medium is injected directly into a coronary artery and the blood is for a short period of time replaced by the contrast medium. This gives a high iodine concentration, enabling selective coronary angiography to reveal small details of the vessels. There is a risk attached to exchanging the physiological blood with the highly unphysiological contrast medium solution. Apart from its content of contrast medium molecules, the solution differs from blood in several respects: it has often a higher osmolality, it does not contain all the electrolytes of blood, it

Dept of Diagnostic Radiology, Malmö General Hospital, University of Lund, S-21401 Malmö, Sweden

Frontiers in European Radiology, Vol. 8
Eds. Baert/Heuck
© Springer-Verlag, Berlin Heidelberg 1991

has per volume unit a lower content of oxygen molecules than arterial blood, and it carries less oxygen to the tissues of the body.

In arteriography the only desirable contrast medium effect is attenuation of radiation. All other effects are regarded as adverse, and these adverse effects may be related in a simplified way, to three factors:

1. The chemotoxicity of the contrast medium molecule (binding to enzymes and other proteins, effects on cell membranes and cell organelles, release of vasoactive substances)
2. Osmotoxicity (movement of water across cell membranes due to the restricted passage of the contrast media through the membranes)
3. Toxic effects of the contrast medium solvent (nonoptimal electrolyte concentrations, pH, oxygen content, and carbon dioxide content)

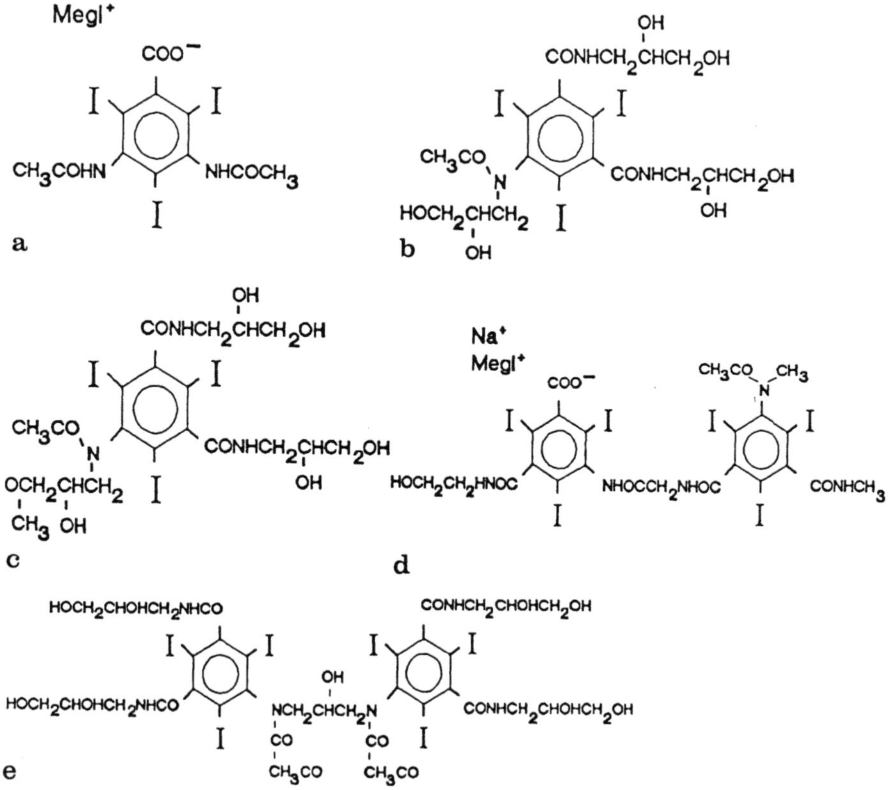

Fig. 1 a–e. Chemical structures of radiographic contrast media: **a** diatrizoate (ionic monomer), **b** iohexol (nonionic monomer), **c** iopentol (nonionic monomer), **d** ioxaglate (ionic dimer), and **e** iodixanol (nonionic dimer)

In the 1930s it was found that the X-ray attenuating iodine atom could be incorporated into a benzene ring derivative; the group of *ionic high osmolar monomeric contrast media* (Fig. 1a) [82]. The benzene ring is the anion and contains one COO^--group. Initially sodium (Na^+) was used as the only cation. The contrast media had a comparatively low chemotoxicity but still had negative effects (effects, for instance, on the formation and conduction of electrical impulses in the heart, the effect of reducing myocardial contractile force (CF), and vasodilatatory and rheologic effects). In order to obtain an adequate iodine concentration, the amount of sodium had to be high. This has a disadvantage in that a higher frequency of ventricular fibrillation (VF) is produced by media with high sodium concentrations, at the level of $90\,mM$ Na^+ at $350\,mg$ I/ml [90]. The contrast medium toxicity is thus not only related to the iodine-carrying benzene ring and osmolality, but also to the sodium ion. These ionic monomers also had a comparatively low water solubility. By exchanging sodium for the organic cation meglumine an increased water solubility was achieved as well as an increased lethal dose for 50% of the group (LD_{50}) [6]. A drawback was that if most of the sodium was exchanged with meglumine, especially with sodium concentrations lower than $60\,mM$ Na^+, there was increased risk of cardiac arrhythmias and VF [78]. It is thought, therefore, that, both experimentally and clinically, ionic monomeric contrast media cause the lowest frequency of adverse effects on the heart if the sodium concentration is close to the physiological level, i.e., about $150\,mM$ Na^+ [70, 85].

To decrease the risk of adverse effects from the ionic contrast media, cations other than sodium and meglumine have been investigated. A small amount of calcium reduces both the risk of VF and the medium's negative influence on CF [75]. Furthermore, tolerance of the contrast medium increases if a small amount of magnesium is added, i.e., LD_{50} increases.

Ionic monomeric contrast media thus consist of a radiopaque anion and a non-radiopaque cation. This creates a much higher osmolality than the 290 mosmol/kg of plasma. At iodine concentrations used in coronary angiography (300–370 mg/ml) the osmolality is 1500–2000 mosmol/kg [30]. Such high osmolality draws water out of the red blood cells and vascular endothelium, dilates blood vessels, and produces pain [1, 2]. As the anion contains three iodine atoms, the ratio of the number of iodine atoms to the number of contrast medium particles (molecules or ions) in an ideal solution is $3:2 = 1.5$.

It was suggested by *Almén* in 1969 that, in order to reduce osmolality contrast media which do not dissociase into cations and anions should be synthesized [1]. The group of *nonionic monomeric contrast media* contains a radiopaque molecule with three iodine atoms (Fig. 1b, c). The molecule has several polar hydroxyl groups to create the water solubility. The ratio of iodine atoms to contrast medium particles in an ideal solution is higher ($3:1 = 3$) than that of the ionic contrast media ($3:2 = 1.5$). The osmolality of the nonionic monomeric contrast media is 600–860 mosmol/kg at iodine concentrations of 300–370 mg/ml [30, 36].

To provide another way of reducing contrast medium osmolality, an ionic ratio 3 contrast medium, ioxaglate, has been synthesized (Fig. 1d). Ioxaglate is an *ionic (monoacidic) dimer* consisting of a radiopaque anion which has one negatively charged carboxyl group ($-COO^+$) and one accompanying cation. The anion contains two benzene ring derivatives with a total of six iodine atoms. As the cation is not radiopaque, the ratio of iodine atoms to contrast medium particles in an ideal solution is $6:2 = 3$, which is the same as for the nonionic monomers [84]. The cations of ioxaglate are meglumine and sodium. Ioxaglate has a slightly lower osmolality (600 mosmol/kg with 320 mg I/ml) than the nonionic monomers but a higher chemotoxicity [22, 30].

The osmolality of a contrast medium can be further reduced by synthesizing molecular dimers of two benzoic acid derivatives which do not dissociate (Fig. 1e). The group of *nonionic dimers* contains a total of six iodine atoms in which hydroxyl groups create the water solubility [23]. The ratio of iodine atoms to contrast medium particles in an ideal solution is $6:2 = 6$. The low osmolalities of the nonionic dimers have made it necessary to add osmotically active substances to the media in order to reach the osmolality of plasma.

Both in the normal [39, 40, 42, 85] and ischemic heart [29, 33, 76] these new groups of contrast agents cause a significantly lower frequency of adverse effects than the high osmolar media (less influence on heart rate, blood flow, drop of blood pressure, CF, ECG changes, arrhythmias, VF, cardiac arrest, and death). The lower frequency of adverse effects occurs in spite of the absence of the ions of plasma (concerning the nonionic media) or with the cationic content as in the high osmolar media (concerning ioxaglate). This is probably the reason why the interest in investigating additions of cations to low osmolar contrast media has been small.

In spite of their advantages, the nonionic contrast media still have undesirable effects such as, for example, ECG changes, arrhythmias and angina pectoris pain [44]. The media also cause some deaths [21, 51, 89]. The highest mortality rate is found among patients with advanced cardiac disease, and it is especially important to reduce undesirable effects among these people, who are often old and frail. As has been said, the sodium content of the ionic contrast media is important in reducing adverse effects of these media on the heart. A proper sodium concentration is especially important in reducing influence on the electrical conduction of the heart, and causes fewer ECG changes, arrhythmias and VFs. There is thus the possibility that if sodium is added to the nonionic contrast media, it might further reduce the adverse effects from these media.

Ischemic changes during cardioangiography and coronary angiography have been found clinically (ECG changes with ST-segment depression, angina pectoris pain) [31, 38, 44]. The nonionic monomeric contrast medium iopamidol tends to increase myocardial oxygen consumption [34]. On the other hand, experimental investigations have often produced conflicting results, and contrast media have not been considered to gain from being saturated with oxygen [31, 85, 86]. It is thus important to investigate further whether creating a more physiological oxygenated contrast medium could be beneficial.

During conventional cardioangiography, contrast media are injected at concentrations of 300–370 mg I/ml. In the past decade, digital subtraction angiography (DSA) has become increasingly popular. In DSA, lower concentrations (e.g., 140–160 mg I/ml) of contrast media may be used [62, 63]. This might cause an altered risk from the media. Concerning the high osmolar contrast media, a reduction, for instance to 140 mg I/ml, causes a more pronounced decrease in osmolality than is caused by the low osmolar monomers. This could change the relative importance of adverse effects from the contrast media as well as the importance of those from a sodium addition.

Most experimental cardioangiographic investigations are performed using hearts from animals free from disease, which is in contradiction to the clinical situation. In order to imitate a clinical situation, investigations should be performed not only during normal perfusion pressure but also during ischemic conditions with reduced pressure.

If it were possible to achieve a contrast medium with an osmolality equal to blood (about 300 mosmol/kg) with the electrolytes of blood (where sodium is the most common ion) and saturated with oxygen, a better, more physiological contrast medium could be used in cardioangiography and selective coronary angiography. To address this problem a series of investigations was performed in the isolated rabbit heart [8–12]. The investigations were aimed especially at answering the following questions:

1. What are the fibrillatory propensities and influences on CF of monomeric and dimeric ionic and nonionic contrast media in the isolated rabbit heart?
2. Does enrichment of nonionic monomeric contrast media with NaCl and/or oxygen reduce the risk of VF or other arrhythmias during normal and ischemic conditions?
3. Does enrichment of nonionic monomeric contrast media with NaCl and/or oxygen have a beneficial effect on CF during normal and ischemic conditions?

2 Materials and Methods

Rabbits of both sexes (Swedish Land) were anesthetized i.v. with pentobarbitone (Mebumal Vet., ACO) and heparinized (Heparin, Kabi Vitrum, 1000 IU/kg). Through a sternal incision, the heart was removed en bloc and mounted in the ascending aorta on a cannula according to the Langendorff technique [47]. For perfusion of the hearts Krebs' solution was used. The Krebs' solution contained 118 mM NaCl, 24.9 mM NaHCO$_3$, 2.52 mM CaCl$_2$, 4.69 mM KCl, 1.18 mM KH$_2$PO$_4$ and 1.16 mM MgSO$_4$. To this solution was added 11.0 mM glucose and 12.0 mM sucrose [57]. When the coronary perfusion had started, the pulmonary artery was incised to permit optimal drainage from the heart and obtain samples for oxygen tension measurements.

The experimental system is given in Fig. 2. The perfusion fluid of Krebs' solution was stored in a glass container where it was saturated with a mixture of 95% oxygen and 5% carbon dioxide. From the container the perfusion fluid was delivered through two parallel plastic tubes connected with a T valve to the aortic cannula just above its entrance into the aorta. The T valve was turned so that the connection between one of the plastic tubes and the aortic catheter was closed. Contrast medium solution was then injected into the closed tube while perfusion fluid simultaneously flowes through the other tube. Then the T valve was turned so

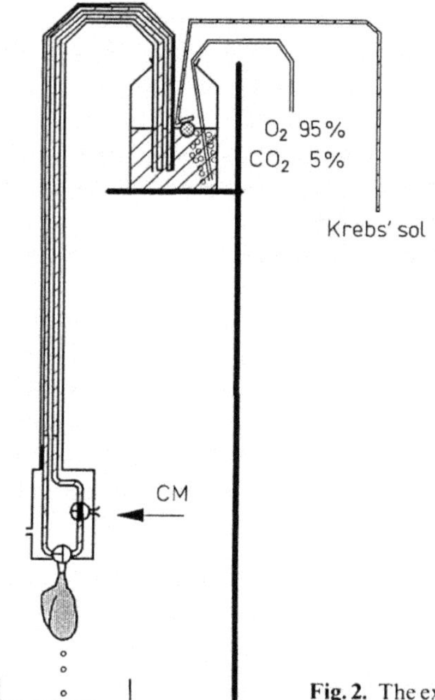

Fig. 2. The experimental Langendorff system used for perfusing isolated rabbit hearts. *CM*, contrast medium

that the flow of perfusion fluid to the aortic catheter was stopped and the flow of contrast medium solution was started. If VF occurred, the T valve made it possible to stop the fibrillation by exchanging the flow of contrast medium solution for perfusion fluid. The heart preparation was therefore, presumably, protected from damage due to prolonged fibrillation.

For measurement of the CF a strain gauge (Dept of Medical Technology, Malmö General Hospital) was sutured to the wall of the left ventricle. For studying VF, needle electrodes for ECG were placed into the remnants of the mediastinal tissue behind the heart. A Mingograph 800 (Elema Schönander, Sweden) was used for recordings of CF and ECG.

During investigations in which only *normal* perfusion pressure was used, the pressure of perfusion fluid and contrast medium solutions was 75–80 cm H_2O. During investigations in which *reduced* pressure was also used, the perfursion was carried out at two standard positions. One was the *normal* perfusion pressure of 75 cm H_2O, and the other a *reduced* perfusion pressure of 35 cm H_2O. At *reduced* pressure the heart was perfused for 5 min before infusing the contrast medium solution. After the contrast medium solution had passed the heart, or after VF had occurred, the heart was perfused at *normal* pressure. If the next contrast medium infusion was to be performed at *normal* pressure, the heart was allowed to rest for 10 min. If it was to be performed at *reduced* pressure, the heart was allowed to rest for 7 min at *normal* before the pressure was reduced. The heart was

Table 1. Details of investigation series

Series	Contrast medium	Concetration (mg I/ml)	No. of hearts	Volume infused (ml)	mM NaCl	Oxygen	Reduced pressure	Investigation	Corresponding figure in the text
1	Meglumine diatrizoate Iopentol Equimolor glucose	140 140 —	35	20	0, 77, 154	Without	Without	VF, CF	3, 7
2[a]	Iohexol Iopentol	350 350	15 15	7.5 7.5	0, 10, 20 0, 10, 20	Without Without	Without Without	VF VF	 4
3[b]	Iohexol Iohexol	350	15	7.5	10, 20 10, 20	Without	Without	VF	
4	Iohexol	350	16	5	0, 28	Without	Without/with	VF	
5	Iohexol	350	10	7.5	0, 10	Without/with	Without	VF	
6	Iohexol	350	10	7.5	—	Without/with	Without/with	VF	
7	Iohexol Iodixanol Ioxaglate	 320	 15	 9	0, 20 24 155	Without	Without	VF, CF	 5, 6
8	Iohexol	150	15	7.5	0, 19.3, 38.5 57.8, 77, 154	Without	Without	CF	8
9	Iopentol	350	15	5	0, 19.3, 38.5, 57.8, 77	Without	Without	CF	9
10	Iohexol Iopentol	300	15	5	0, 29, 77	Without	Without	CF	
11	Iohexol Ioxaglate	160	10	10	—	Without/with	Without	CF	10
12	Iohexol	150	16	7.5	—	Without/with	Without/with	CF	
13	Iohexol	150	16	7.5	0, 28	Without/with	With	CF	11

VF, ventricular fibrillation; CF, contractile force. [a]The order to the hearts was redomized in both of these series.
[b] Sodium was added as NaCl or as the salts of Krebs' solution, with the other electrolytes of Krebs' solution corresponding to the NaCl concentration.

then perfused at reduced pressure for 5 min before the contrast medium infusion. The contrast medium solutions were infused at 37°C.

Oxygenation was achieved with the contrast medium solution bubbled for 5 min with 100% oxygen at 37°C (0.5 1 O_2/min) immediately before the infusion into the heart. An amount of contrast medium solution corresponding to one infusion was oxygenated at each instance.

The contrast media used were:

- Meglumine diatrizoate (Angiografin, Schering AG)—a ratio 1.5, high osmolar, ionic monomeric contrast medium.
- Iohexol (Omnipaque, Nycomed A/S)—a ratio 3, low osmolar, nonionic monomeric contrast medium.
- Iopentol (Nycomed A/S)—a ratio 3, low osmolar, nonionic monomeric contrast medium which is under clinical investigation [16].
- Sodium/meglumine ioxaglate (Hexabrix, Laboratoire Guerbet)—a ratio 3, low osmolar, monoacidic dimer.
- Iodixanol (Nycomed A/S)—a ratio 6, low osmolar, nonionic dimer which is under clinical investigation.
- A glucose solution, equimolar to meglumine diatrizoate and iopentol 140 mg I/ml was used.

The investigation series performed are given in Table 1.

Wilcoxon's signed rank test was used for statistical analyses of CF. The fourfold table test with Yates' correction was used for statistical analysis of VF. A p value less than 0.05 was considered significant. The words "statistically significant" and "significant" will be used with the same meaning.

3 Results

3.1 Ventricular Fibrillation

When increasing concentrations of NaCl were added to meglumine diatrizoate (140 mg I/ml) and iopentol (140 mg I/ml) the frequency of VF decreased (series 1, Fig. 3). Diatrizoate without sodium caused the highest frequency of VF. Even if not statistically significant, there was a tendency for the nonionic medium iopentol *without* sodium to cause a higher frequency of VF than the ionic medium diatrizoate *with* sodium. An equimolar glucose solution caused no VF, but when infused without sodium it caused asystolia in four hearts.

When increasing concentrations of NaCl were added to iohexol (350 mg I/ml) or iopentol (350 mg I/ml) the number of VFs decreased (series 2a, and b, Fig. 4). Without sodium both contrast media caused 15/15 VFs, with 20 mM NaCl iohexol caused 1/15 VFs while iopentol caused 0/15 VFs. An intermediate number of VFs was caused by 10 mM NaCl. No difference was found between the two contrast media at equal sodium concentrations.

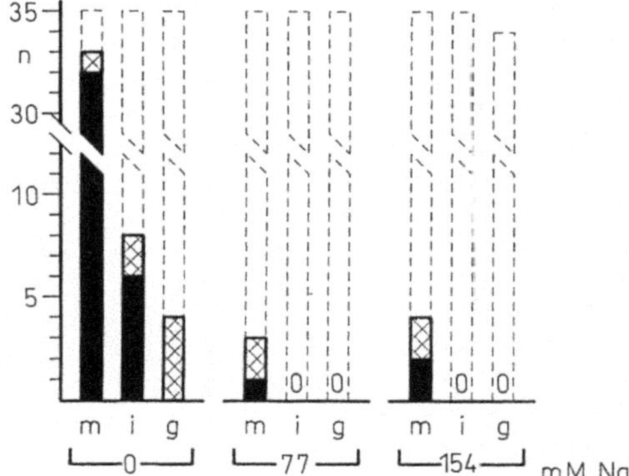

Fig. 3 Ventricular fibrillation (■) and asystoles (▨) after infusion of 20 ml meglumine diatrizoate (140 mg I/ml); (*m*), iopentol (140 mg I/ml); (*i*), or glucose (0.37 *M*); (*g*) with 0, 77 or 154 m*M* Na⁺ (35 hearts)

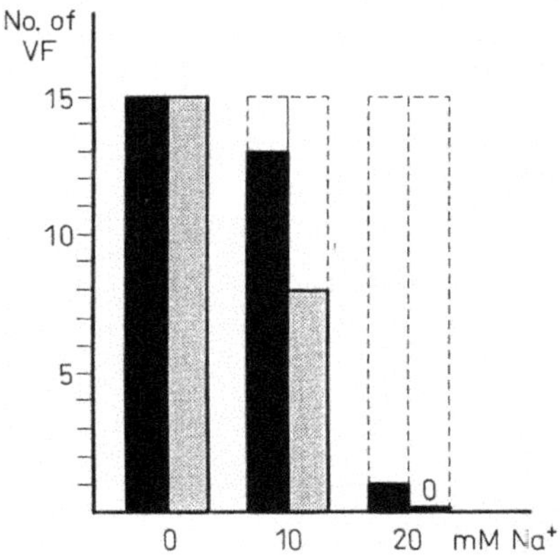

Fig 4. The number of ventricular fibrillations (*VF*) after infusing 7.5 ml iohexol (350 mg I/ml) (■) or 7.5 ml iopentol (350 mg I/ml) (▨) with 0, 10 or 20 m*M* NaCl (15 hearts)

Iohexol (350 mg I/ml) caused a lower frequency of VFs when 20 m*M* Na⁺ were added as NaCl or as *Krebs' solution* salts (series 3). No difference was found between adding Na⁺ as NaCl and as Krebs' solution salts.

Iohexol (350 mg I/ml) was infused during *normal* and *reduced* perfusion pressure with 0 or 28 m*M* NaCl (series 4). Iohexol without NaCl caused a higher frequency of VF than were caused with 28 m*M* NaCl. This was found both during normal and reduced pressure. No difference was found between the two sodium concentrations when compared at equal perfusion pressures.

Iohexol (350 mg I/ml) without sodium caused a higher frequency of VFs than when infused with 10 m*M* NaCl both without and with *oxygen saturation* (series 5). Oxygen was found to exert no influence on the frequency of VFs. Iohexol (350 mg I/ml) was injected during *normal* and *reduced* perfusion pressure, without and with *oxygen saturation* (series 6). The frequency of VFs was unchanged when iohexol was saturated with oxygen.

Iohexol (320 mg I/ml), iodixanol (320 mg I/ml) and ioxaglate (320 mg I/ml) were infused into 15 hearts (series 7, Fig. 5). Iohexol without sodium caused the highest

                                                    L. Bååth

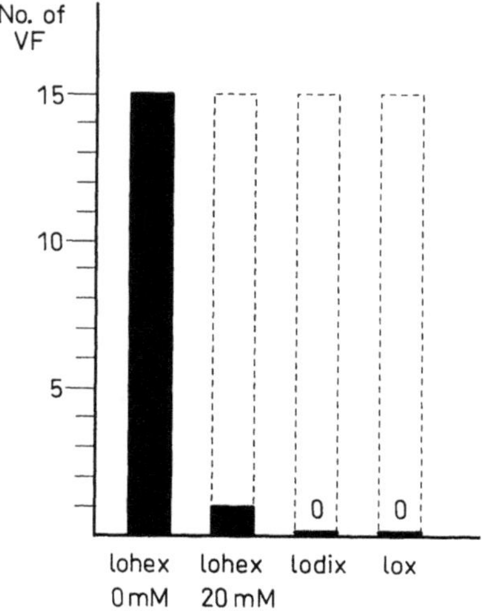

Fig. 5. The number of ventricular fibrillation (VF) after infusing 9 ml iohexol (Iohex; 320 mg I/ml) with 0 or 20 mM Na$^+$, iodixanol (Iodix; 320 mg I/ml) and sodium/meglumine ioxaglate (Iox; 320 mg I/ml) (15 hearts)

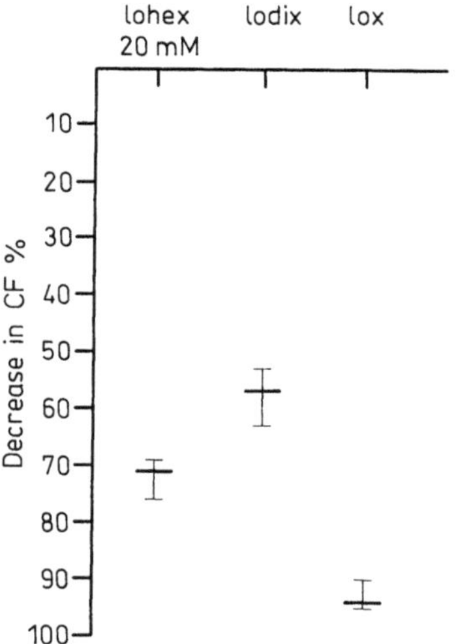

Fig. 6. Decrease in contractile force when infusing 9 ml iohexol (320 mg I/ml) with 20 mM Na$^+$ (14 hearts), iodixanol (320 mg I/ml, 15 hearts) and sodium/meglumine ioxaglate (320 mg I/ml, 15 hearts) (median and interquartile range)

frequency of VFs, 15/15, which was reduced to 1/15 when 20 mM NaCl was added. Iodixanol (containing 24 mM NaCl) and ioxaglate (containing 155 mM NaCl) caused no VFs. In the hearts where VF did not occur the contractile force was calculated (Fig. 6). Iodixanol caused the smallest influence on CF while ioxaglate caused the most pronounced. Iohexol with 20 mM NaCl caused an intermediate influence on CF (iohexol without sodium caused VF in all hearts, so CF could not be calculated).

3.2 Contractile Force

In series 1, meglumine diatrizoate (140 mg I/ml), iopentol (140 mg I/ml) and an equimolar glucose solution were infused. The number of VFs has been presented above. CF was measured in the hearts where VF or asystolia did not occur (or where very weak CF before infusion made measurements impossible) (Fig. 7). Diatrizoate caused the most pronounced influence on VF, glucose the smallest. Concerning both iopentol and glucose, the smallest influence on CF was found when 77 mM NaCl was added.

Iohexol (150 mg I/ml) was added with increasing concentrations of NaCl (0–154 mM) (series 8, Fig. 8). The smallest influence on CF was found when 19.3 mM NaCl were added. Also, when increasing concentrations of sodium were added to iopentol (350 mg I/ml) the smallest influence on CF was found with concentrations

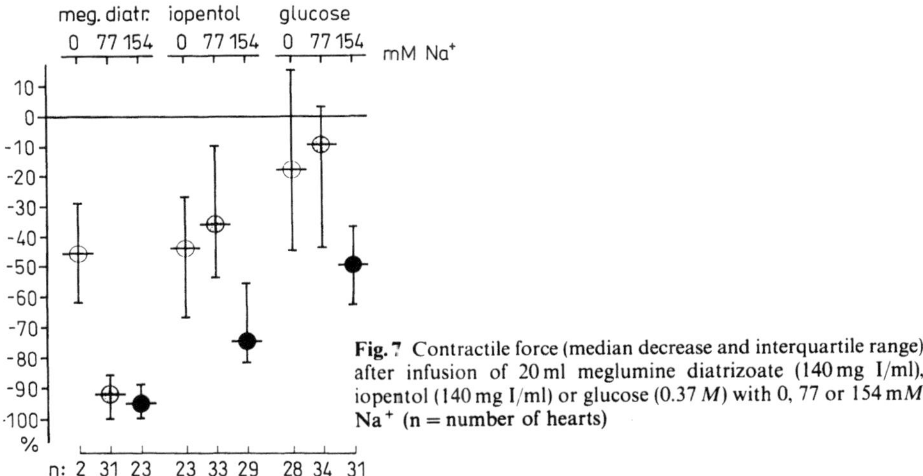

Fig. 7 Contractile force (median decrease and interquartile range) after infusion of 20 ml meglumine diatrizoate (140 mg I/ml), iopentol (140 mg I/ml) or glucose (0.37 M) with 0, 77 or 154 mM Na$^+$ (n = number of hearts)

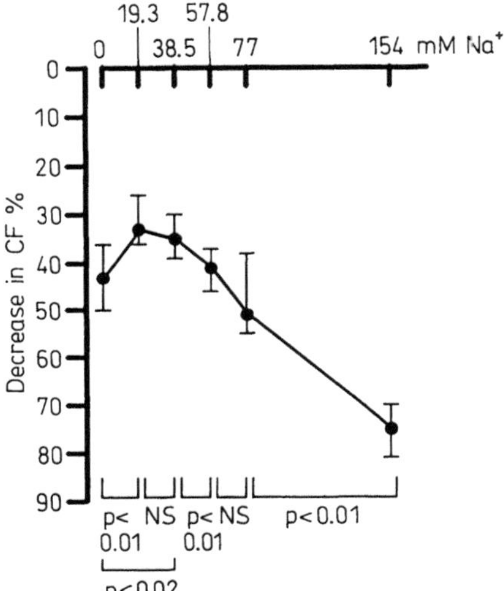

Fig. 8. Contractile force (*CF*; median decrease and interquartile range) after infusion of 7.5 ml iohexol (150 mg I/ml) with 0, 19.3, 38.5, 57.8, 77 or 154 mM Na$^+$ (15 hearts)

at the level of 19.3–38.5 mM NaCl (series 9, Fig. 9). Comparable results were found when iohexol (300 mg I/ml) and iopentol (300 mg I/ml) were used (series 10).

When iohexol (160 mg I/ml) and sodium meglumine ioxaglate (160 mg I/ml) were infused without and with *oxygen saturation*, the smallest influence on CF was found with oxygen (series 11, Fig. 10). Iohexol (150 mg I/ml) without and with *oxygen saturation* was infused both during *normal* and *reduced* perfusion pressure (series 12, Fig 10). During both pressures a lower influence on CF was found with oxygen saturation than without. The influence on CF from the contrast medium was most pronounced during reduced pressure.

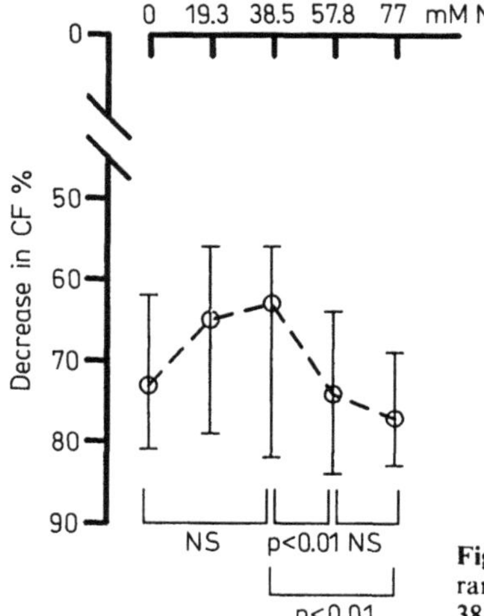

Fig. 9 Contractile force (*CF*; median decrease and interquartile range) after infusion of 5 ml iopentol (350 mg I/ml) with 0, 19.3, 38.5, 57.8 or 77 mM Na⁺ (13 hearts). *NS*, not significant

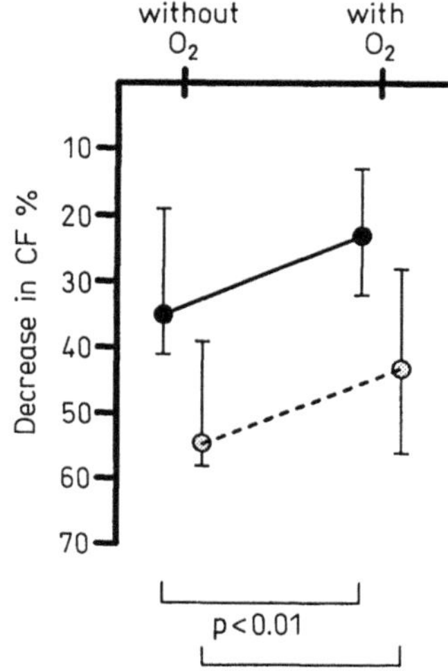

Fig 10. Contractile force (*CF*; median decrease and interquartile range) after infusing 10 ml iohexol (160 mg I/ml) or sodium/meglumine ioxaglate (160 mg/ml). The contrast medium solutions were infused without and with oxygen saturation (10 hearts). *Solid line,* iohexol, *broken line,* ioxaglate

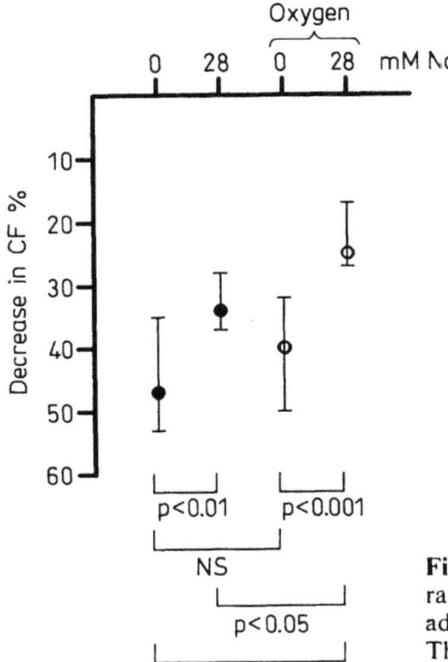

Fig. 11. Contractile force (CF; median decrease and interquartile range) after infusing 7.5 ml iohexol (150 mg I/ml), without sodium addition or with NaCl 28 mM without or with oxygen saturation. The contrast medium solutions were infused during reduced (35 cm H_2O) perfusion pressure (16 hearts)

Iohexol (150 mg I/ml) without sodium and oxygen caused a more pronounced influence on CF than with 28 mM NaCl or with oxygen alone (series 13, Fig. 11). When both 28 mM NaCl *and* oxygen were added, the smallest influence on CF was found. All infusions were performed during reduced perfusion pressure.

4 Discussion

4.1 Electrophysiologic Aspects

In order to understand the important of sodium addition to nonionic contrast media, it is necessary to consider the electrophysiologic aspects of the conduction of impulses and the contractility of the heart.

The electrophysiologic events during the cardiac cycle are divided in phases (phases 0 to 4). It is simplest to start by describing phase 4, the resting potential; during this phase the permeability of potassium is high through the sarcolemma, causing a passive outflow of this ion. The intracellular potassium concentration is about 150 mM. To maintain the intracellular K^+ concentration there is an active, ATP-dependent, inward movement of K^+ across the sarcolemma in return for sodium (the Na/K pump) [24]. The permeability through the sarcolemma is low for sodium, calcium, and chloride, so the transmembrane resting potential is to the greatest extent determined by the concentration gradient of potassium over the cell membrane [43]. The interior of the cell is negative compared to the outside, the resting potential being in the range $- 80$ to $- 95$ mV.

When an excitatory current reaches the sarcolemma, or when the threshold level is reached spontaneously, there is an opening of fast sodium channels and an influx of sodium [43]. The permeability of potassium decreases. This creates a fast, inwardly directed current and the "rapid depolarization" phase (phase 0). The depolarization of the sarcolemma initiates systole of the heart. The transmembrane potential during phase 0 is to the greatest extent determined by the concentration gradient of sodium over the cell membrane. At the peak of the depolarization the potential will reach about + 20 mV. The sodium channels close after 1 to 2 ms [55].

Depolarization is followed by the "early repolarization" phase (phase 1). This phase is believed to occur through closing of the sodium channels and an inward movement of a small amount of potassium.

During phase 0 also an inwardly directed current begins which to the greatest extent is carried by calcium [45, 68]. This is called a "slow current" and this "slow response" is caused by the opening of "slow" calcium channels and lasts until the end of phase 3. The "slow" channels are specific passive calcium channels [87]. The decreased permeability of potassium and the influx of calcium prevents a fall in the membrane potential. This creates a sustained depolarization (the "plateau" phase, phase 2) which lasts over 100 ms [14]. The influx of calcium initiates the release of calcium bound in the sarcoplasmatic reticulum (SR). Calcium from these extra- and intracellular sources is used for contraction of the myofibrils [25, 27, 50].

Phase 2 ends when the permeability of potassium returns to the high level of the resting cell, the repolarization phase (phase 3). The brings the transmembrane potential down to the resting potential of − 80 mV (phase 4). During repolarization, calcium from the myofibrils is pumped back to SR [27]. Calcium is also transported out from the cell via exchange with sodium from the outside of the cell, the Na/Ca-exchange [64, 72]. The Na/Ca-exchange mechanism causes the exchange of one calcium ion in return for three sodium ions [71]. The exchange can take place in both directions depending on the concentration gradient for sodium [64]. The amount of calcium which enters the cell during a cardiac cycle is small, and probably insufficient to activate the myofilaments. Instead, it acts primarily as a trigger to release the calcium bound in SR.

The total sodium concentration in the myocyte is about 30 mM [54]. The concentration of ionized sodium is lower, 6–10 mM, but is not homogeneously distributed in the cell [52]. The concentration of ionized sodium ought to be somewhat higher near the sarcolemma where the sodium exchange takes place.

VF is a choatic asynchronous activity of the heart muscle cells [81]. It is considered to be caused by an abnormally show electrical conduction through the myocardium, or a unidirectional block, causing a re-entry mechanism with a circus movement of pathological impulses [32, 59, 91].

The response from the intracoronary injection of a contrast medium may cause a unidirectional block and a delay in repolarization in a part of the myocardium. A re-entry mechanism could be initiated with a risk of VF [56]. Also, an increased risk of VF is caused by differences in the refractory periods between contrast medium perfused and normal myocardium. Selective injection of a contrast medium solution into one coronary artery, instead of both, is believed to increase the risk of VF [40].

On the cellular level, contrast media can increase the risk of VF via different mechanisms. Ionic contrast media in Tyrodes' solution (i.e., a solution with electrolytes) were found to inactivate the fast sodium channels [58]. The inwardly directed current was carrid through the "slow" calcium channels causing a "slow response". During "slow response" depolarization the action potential is carried through the myocardium at much lower speed than normally [93]. This unnatural depolarization may cause a re-entry mechanism and thus is believed to be associated with an increased risk of arrhythmias and VF [13]. The inhibition of the fast sodium channels was attributed to the chemotoxicity of ionic contrast media. A risk of VF also occurs when the Purkinje fibers depolarize spontaneoulsy. This has been found when the inward current is only carried though the "slow" calcium channels [7, 13].

If the myocardium is perfused with a sodium-free, calcium-containing, solution, no sodium is available to move into the cell, and the fast sodium channels are inactivated [7]. In these circumstances, the inward current is carried through the "slow" calcium channels, causing a "slow response" and a risk of VF [20]. These conditions are present during injections with ionic or nonionic contrast media without sodium. Although the media may lack both sodium and calcium, calcium stored in the basement membrane can be involved in causing the "slow response."

For the control of the contractile force of the myocardium two mechanisms are responsible. One is the classic Frank-Starling response where CF is dependent on the resting length of the cell [80]. The other mechanism is one in which the CF is regulated by the amount of calcium reaching the myofilaments [19, 48, 74]. This in turn is dependent on the concentration of free calcium in the sarcoplasm $[Ca]_i$. The amount of calcium reaching the sarcoplasm is dependent on the cell's ionic environment, $[Ca]_o$, which is the interstitial fluid and, more precisely, the basement membrane of the sarcolemma [41, 49]. Calcium is also stored in SR and in the mitochondria [18, 26]. At depolarization the calcium from the basement membrane enters the sarcoplasm. Calcium enters partly through the "slow channels" and partly via exchange with sodium in the cell, Na/Ca-exchange. There are also hormonal and pharmacological influences on the sarcolemma and on the myofilaments [77].

An increase in $[Ca]_o$ causes an increase in $[Ca]_i$ (via "slow channels" or Na/Ca-exchange). An increase in $[Ca]_i$, directly, and through mediating calcium release from SR, causes an increase in CF [19]. There is a competition between Na^+ and Ca^{2+} for transport across the sarcolemma [48]. A decrease in $[Na]_o$, i.e., a decrease in the sodium activity gradient $(\alpha[Na]_o/\alpha[Na]_i)$, augments the calcium influx via the Na/Ca-exchange (the sodium ion activity, $\alpha[Na]$, means effective concentration of the ion) [53]. Thus a decrease in $[Na]_o$ will produce an increase in $[Ca]_i$ with an increase in CF. A change in the sodium activity gradient has little or no effect on the amount of calcium passing through the "slow channels".

4.2 Contrast Media and Ventricular Fibrillation

The optimal amount of sodium in an ionic monomeric contrast medium has been approximated to about the physiological level, $150\,mM$ Na^+. This is also the sodium content of the monoacidic dimer ioxaglate at 320 mg I/ml. Nonionic monomeric contrast media have not been thought to benefit from the addition of electrolytes [86]. On the other hand, Morris et al. found that a mixture of equal volumes of iohexol (76 mg I/ml) and sodium diatrizoate (140 mg I/ml) caused a lower frequency of VFs than iohexol (140 mg I/ml) without sodium [62]. An intact dog heart model with prolonged coronary infusions was used. Sodium diatrizoate (140 mg I/ml) contains 168 mM Na$^+$. Most probably, the reduced frequency of VFs in the mixture of iohexol and diatrizoate was caused by the sodium content. For further investigations of sodium additions to nonionic contrast media it is preferable to use an anion (chloride) with fewer adverse effects than the anionic benzene ring of an ionic contrast medium. In the present investigations, therefore, sodium was added, mainly in the form of NaCl.

When the heart is infused with an electrolyte-free solution, the lack of sodium causes the depolarization of the cells to be performed through the "slow" sodium channels. This causes the risk of arrhythmias. With a contrast medium solution, the risk is aggravated by the solution's chemotoxicity, which inhibits fast channels and also cause "slow channel" depolarization [58]. Mannitol, which in this context can be considered nontoxic, does not inhibit the fast sodium channels and does not create "slow response." In series I (Fig. 3) an equimolar glucose solution was infused in addition to the contrast media. Glucose may be considered to have similar effects on the heart to those of mannitol, and this may be the reason why the glucose infusions did not cause any VFs. Reflecting a comparatively pronounced chemotoxic effect, the ionic meglumine diatrizoate (0–154 mM Na$^+$) caused the highest frequency of VF, while iopentol (0–154 mM Na$^+$), with a lower chemotoxic effect, caused a smaller number of VFs.

Iopentol (140 mg I/ml) without sodium showed a tendency to a higher frequency of VFs than diatrizoate with 77 or 154 mM Na$^+$ and a higher frequency of VFs than the equimolar glucose solution with 0–154 mM Na$^+$ (Fig. 3). The higher frequency of VFs from iopentol (140 mg I/ml) without sodium than from diatrizoate with 77 or 154 mM Na$^+$ is not in agreement with the results of investigations at *high* iodine concentration [3, 39, 85]. In those investigations nonionic contrast media (without sodium) were found less likely to cause VFs than ionic monomeric contrast media (with sodium). The different results in the present investigation are probably due to the low concentrations and osmolalities of the media. At *high* concentrations, with higher chemotoxicities and osmotoxicities of the ionic monomer, the fibrillation-protective effect from sodium is not sufficient to give the ionic monomer a lower frequency of VFs than an nonionic monomer without sodium. At *low* concentrations the fibrillation-protective effect from sodium will be relatively stronger. The ionic monomer with sodium thereby causes a lower frequency of VFs than the nonionic monomer without sodium.

These findings indicated that sodium reduced the risk of VF not only for ionic monomeric contrast media, but also for nonionic monomeric contrast media. The highest increase in protection against VF occurred when the sodium content in the test solutions was somewhere between 0 and 77 mM. It was therefore of interest to find out whether a smaller addition of sodium caused a significant reduction in the frequency of VF from a nonionic monomeric contrast medium. The reason for this was that, according to previous physiological investigations, sodium causes a negative inotropic effect [17, 46, 53].

When 10–28 mM Na$^+$ were added to iohexol and iopentol (350 mg I/ml) in the present investigation the risk of VF was significantly reduced. These sodium additions were considerably lower than what is considered necessary for high osmolar ionic contrast media. For those media, a fibrillation- protective effect has only been found from adding 45–190 mM Na$^+$, while 0–40 mM Na$^+$ caused a high frequency of VF [78]. Thus, reflecting the lower chemo- and osmotoxicities of nonionic monomeric contrast media, it is sufficient with a considerably smaller sodium addition to the nonionic media, to gain a fibrillation-protective effect. In the present investigation series, as well as in several series not published, no VF has occurred when an amount equal to or less than 30 mM NaCl has been added to nonionic contrast media. In the dog, sodium additions as low as about 3 mM Na$^+$ have decreased the risk of VF [37, 61].

The reduced fibrillation frequency brought about by adding 45–190 mM Na$^+$ to ionic high osmolar contrast media was attributed to a prolongation of phases 2 and 3 of the cardiac cycle, which caused a prolongation of the refractory period of the cell [78]. The fibrillation-protective effect from adding 10–28 mM Na$^+$ to nonionic contrast media may also the attributed to this prolongation of the refractory period. Besides, the small additions of sodium may be sufficient to maintain the action potential by the fast sodium channels. Thereby the "slow response" action potential, caused by lack of sodium, will be counteracted.

Ions other than sodium may be added to contrast media. The addition of small amounts of *calcium* to ionic contrast media reduces the frequency of VF during *normal* perfusion pressure [65, 83, 94]. All electrolytes in Krebs' solution were added to a nonionic contrast medium (iohexol 350 mg I/ml) to find out whether it produced a lower risk of VF than the addition of NaCl (series 3). No difference was found between the addition of a small amount of sodium as NaCl and its addition as the electrolytes of Krebs' solution. However, there may be another composition of NaCl and other electrolytes that, when added to iohexol, reduces the risk of VF more than NaCl alone.

It is of interest to investigate whether the reduced risk of VF from a small addition of sodium is also present during ischemia. This is because, during ischemia, the addition of *calcium* to an ionic monomeric contrast medium has been alleged to cause an increased risk of VF [76]. The positive inotropic effect from calcium addition, during *normal* perfusion pressure, was reversed during ischemia, and this could cause instability between normal and ischemic areas of the heart. The instability was attributed to an imbalance between supply and demand of oxygen and energy-rich substrates during ischemia. A similar instability might be expected if, as in the present investigations, a comparatively positive inotropic effect is produced by adding about 28 mM Na$^+$ to nonionic contrast media. It was found that the reduced risk of VF from adding sodium was the same during both *normal* and *reduced* perfusion pressure and that no negative effects from the sodium addition were found during *reduced* pressure. This indicates that the sodium-related increase in CF does not lead to an imbalance between supply and demand of oxygen and energy-rich substrates in the myocardium.

In selective coronary arteriography there might be less difference in oxygen tension between contrast medium-perfused and blood-perfused myocardium when an oxygenated contrast medium is used. In the arteriosclerotic heart, an oxygenated contrast medium might therefore carry a lower risk of VF. However, it was found that, during both *normal* and *reduced* perfusion pressure, oxygenation of iohexol (350 mg I/ml) did not influence the risk of VF. Iohexol without sodium tended to cause a higher frequency of VF during *reduced* pressure than during *normal* perfusion pressure, but the difference was not significant. In dog hearts, the ventricular fibrillation threshold method (VFT) has shown that both ionic and nonionic contrast media caused a higher fibrillatory propensity during ischemia or early myocardial infarction than during normal perfusion pressure [95]. As both coronary arteries are simultaneously infused in the isolated rabbit heart model, the whole myocardium receives the same perfusion fluid. In coronary arteriosclerosis with different degrees of ischemia in different parts of the myocardium, the associated differences in refractory periods in various regions increase the heart's vulnerability to VF [73].

Even if the introduction of low osmolar contrast media has meant a reduction of chemotoxicities, striking differences concerning the influences on the rabbit heart were found between a nonionic monomer (iohexol), a monoacidic dimer (ioxaglate), and a nonionic dimer (iodixanol); (Fig. 5). Iohexol (320 mg I/ml) without sodium caused VF in all 15 hearts in the investigation series. When 20 mM Na$^+$ was added, iohexol (320 mg I/ml) caused VF in one of 15 hearts. Ioxaglate (320 mg I/ml) and iodixanol (320 mg I/ml, with NaCl 24 mM) caused no VFs. Being an ionic contrast medium, ioxaglate has a higher chemotoxicity than nonionic monomeric contrast media, in spite of a somewhat lower osmolality [23, 79]. Ioxoglate had the most pronounced negative effect on CF (Fig. 6) because it has a higher chemotoxicity and sodium content (150 mM Na$^+$) than iohexol or iodixanol. Ioxaglate's low fibrillatory propensity is therefore probably to a great extent caused by the comparatively high sodium concentration. Iodixanol, which has the lowest osmolality and chemotoxicity [23] caused the smallest influence on CF.

4.3 Contrast Media and Contractile Force

Ionic contrast media usually cause a negative inotropic effect. Nonionic contrast media may cause positive or negative inotropic effects depending on the contrast medium used, the amount and concentration of the contrast medium reaching the myocardium, and the clinical or experimental situation [85]. In the isolated rabbit heart, a negative inotropic effect from both ionic and nonionic media dominates [4, 86].

Sodium is also considered to cause a negative inotropic effect [17, 46, 69]. Thus, with increasing sodium concentrations in a nutrient solution, or in a contrast medium solution, an increased negative inotropic effect is found. In the first investigation series, meglumine diatrizoate, iopentol and glucose were infused with 0, 77 or 154 mM NaCl (Fig. 7). It was expected that the solutions would cause the smallest influence on CF when infused without sodium, and that with the largest NaCl concentration (154 mM), they would cause the greatest influence on CF. It was therefore somewhat puzzling that the smallest influence on CF for both iopentol and glucose was caused when 77 mM NaCl was added. It is remarkable that the beneficial effects of sodium on CF were equal in the iopentol and glucose solutions. Subsequent series were designed to investigate whether there existed an optimal sodium concentration at which the effect on CF was smallest from a nonionic contrast medium solution. The sodium additions ranged from 0 to 154 mM and the smallest effects on CF were found at 20–40 mM Na$^+$.

The fact that the smallest influence on CF was caused by the addition of 20–40 mM Na$^+$ was most probably not due to the changed osmolality of the solutions. Instead, the minimal influence on CF was always in the magnitude of 20–40 mM Na$^+$ independently of the contrast medium concentrations used (150, 300 and 350 mg I/ml). The osmolality of iohexol (350 mg I/ml) is more than double that of iohexol (150 mg I/ml).

The reason why the addition of 20–40 mM Na$^+$ to a nonionic contrast medium causes the smallest influence on CF is unclear, and might be the subject of speculation. When nonionic contrast media with increasing concentrations of sodium (in the range 60–150 mM) pass the extracellular room around the myocardial cell, the increase in sodium activity gradient ($\alpha[\text{Na}]_o/\alpha[\text{Na}]_i$) causes a progressively negative inotropic effect [52]. When the contrast medium is without sodium ions, $\alpha[\text{Na}]_o$ approaches zero. This causes a comparatively lower sodium activity gradient and a more positive inotropic effect. Even if the contrast medium is calcium-free, calcium bound to the basement membrane may be transported inwards via the Na/Ca-exchange mechanism. On the other hand, a zero $\alpha[\text{Na}]_o$ might also cause a sodium efflux from the cell and a decrease in $\alpha[\text{Na}]_i$. This increases the sodium activity gradient ($\alpha[\text{Na}]_o/\alpha[\text{Na}]_i$) and reduces the positive inotropic effect. There might also be an inadequate amount of [Na]$_i$ to participate in a sufficient exchange for [Ca]$_o$.

Enriching the contrast medium with small amounts of sodium (20–40 mM) causes a larger decrease in [Na]$_o$ than enriching with higher sodium concentrations (60–150 mM). The decrease in [Na]$_o$ is smaller than when the sodium-free solution is infused. On the other hand, the sodium efflux from using contrast media with 20–40 mM Na$^+$ instead of 0 mM Na$^+$ might be small, or even absent, because [Na]$_o$ might be close to [Na]$_o$. This might cause a smaller decrease in $\alpha[\text{Na}]_i$. At this level (20–40 mM Na$^+$) there is an adequate amount of [Na]$_i$ to participate in an adequate exchange for [Ca]$_o$. This should result in the most pronounced [Ca]$_i$ causing the strongest contraction of the myofilaments. The optimal sodium concentration, as discussed here, seems to be related to the sodium concentration within the cell.

Oxygen is the first substrate whose supply becomes limited when coronary flow is reduced [60]. In the present investigations, a positive inotropic effect from oxygenation was confined not only to a nonionic monomeric contrast medium. It was also found when ioxaglate (monoacidic dimer) and iodixanol (nonionic dimer) were oxygenated. The effect from oxygen was purely additive, and independent of the use of contrast medium with or without a small addition of sodium.

Ionic monomeric contrast media with sodium and meglumine produce a more pronounced negative inotropic effect during ischemia than during normal perfusion pressure [76, 96]. The more positive inotropic effect from calcium addition to an ionic monomeric contrast medium has been found to be reversed during ischemia [5, 76]. Previous investigations on direct ischemic effects from angiographic contrast media are rare. During angiography of the aorta or of one of its larger branches a generalized lower oxygen pressure has been found in arterial blood [66]. Angina pectoris pain, which is not uncommon during cardioangiography, is also associated with ischemia from the contrast medium [31, 38, 88]. An oxygenated contrast medium solution has not been tried clinically but it might be beneficial in patients with ischemic heart disease. It is therefore important to investigate whether the reduced influence of CF, during *normal* perfusion pressure, from a small amount of sodium and from oxygen saturation, is also present during *reduced* pressure. Addition of $28\,mM$ Na$^+$ as well as oxygenation of iohexol ($150\,mg$ I/ml) reduced the influence on CF during *normal* and *reduced* perfusion pressure. As the *reduced* pressure itself decreased CF this means that the further decrease in CF, caused by contrast medium, was partly counteracted by sodium and oxygen.

The *reduced* perfusion pressure resulted in a lower flow rate of Krebs' solution, and a reduced amount of oxygen was available to the heart. This was reflected in a lower PO$_2$ of Krebs' solution in the pulmonary artery. It might have been expected, therefore, that oxygenation of iohexol would be more beneficial during *reduced* than during *normal* pressure. Contrary to this, the influence from oxygen was additive and the smaller CF from oxygenation was nearly equal during *normal* and *reduced* perfusion pressure. This might mean that already during *normal* pressure the oxygen extraction from iohexol was nearly maximal and that no appreciable extra amount of oxygen was available to the heart during *reduced* pressure. This is in agreement with the measurements of oxygen tension in the Krebs' solution. Before passing the heart, the oxygen tension was about $80\,kPa$. After passing the heart the oxygen tension was $14\,kPa$ during *normal* perfusion pressure and $7\,kPa$ during *reduced* pressure. Therefore the *extra* amount of oxygen utilized during *reduced* perfusion pressure was comparatively small compared to the amount in Krebs' solution before entering the heart. The oxygen consumption of the heart has been found to be lower during *reduced* perfusion pressure [28, 67, 92]. These findings may be the reason why not more than the additive effect from oxygenation was found during *reduced* pressure. On the other hand, in the ischemic heart, with few compensating mechanisms and low CF prior to contrast medium, the oxygenation is probably more important than in the intact heart.

Nonionic monomeric contrast media cause considerably smaller influences on CF than ionic monomeric contrast media. It might therefore seem that the reduced influence on CF, from adding a small amount of sodium or from oxygenation of a nonionic contrast medium, should be without importance. However, the smallest influence on CF should be found when using a contrast medium with *both* a small addition of NaCl *and* oxygen saturation. When an oxygenated iohexol solution ($150\,mg$ I/ml) with $28\,mM$ Na$^+$ was infused, the solution caused about a 50% smaller influence on CF than an iohexol solution without these additions (Fig. 11; infusions during *reduced* perfusion pressure). The same sodium concentration ($28\,mM$ Na$^+$) also significantly reduced the risk of VF. In the ischemic heart, with a reduced contractility and increased vulnerability to arrhythmias, the cardiac effects from the contrast media should be minimized. The addition of a small amount of NaCl (20–40 mM) in combination with oxygen saturation might give a nonionic contrast medium with even smaller adverse effect than those presently used.

5 Summary

It can be concluded from the investigations in the isolated rabbit heart that:

1. At *low* iodine concentrations (140 mg I/ml) the addition of a small amount of sodium as NaCl reduces the risk of VF from ionic and nonionic contrast media. At *high* iodine concentrations (320 and 350 mg I/ml) the addition of a small amount of sodium (20–30 mM Na$^+$), as NaCl or as Krebs' solution salts, reduces the risk of VF from nonionic contrast media.
2. At both *low* and *high* iodine concentrations, the addition of sodium, as NaCl (20–40 mM Na$^+$), to nonionic monomeric contrast media reduces their decrease of CF more than media without sodium and more than media with 60–150 mM NaCl.
3. Oxygen saturation of nonionic monomeric contrast media does not influence the risk of VF from those media.
4. Oxygen saturation of nonionic monomeric and dimeric contrast media, as well as of a monoacidic dimer, reduces their adverse effects on CF.
5. In agreement with the findings during *normal* perfusion pressure, also during *reduced* pressure, the addition of NaCl (10–30 mM Na$^+$) to nonionic monomeric contrast media has two beneficial effects: reduced risk of VF and reduced influence on CF.
6. In agreement with the findings during *normal* pressure, also during *reduced* pressure, oxygen saturation of nonionic monomeric contrast media reduces their adverse effects on contractile force without affecting the risk of VF.
7. Cardiac tolerance of a nonionic monomeric contrast medium, enriched with about 30 mM Na$^+$ as NaCl, and oxygen saturated, could be expected to be still greater than cardiac tolerance of nonionic monomeric media without NaCl and oxygen.

Acknowledgement. The author thanks Ms. Eva Prahl for excellent secretarial assistance.

References

1. Almén T (1969) Contrast agent design. Some aspects on the synthesis of water-soluble contrast agents of low osmolality. J Ther Biol 24:216
2. Almén T (1971) Toxicity of radiocontrast agents. *In*: Knoefel PK (ed) Radiocontrast agents, vol 2. Pergamon Oxford, p 443
3. Almén T (1973) Effects of metrizamide and other contrast media on the isolated rabbit heart. Acta Radiol Suppl (Stockh) 335: 216

4. Almén T, Bååth L (1987) Effects of iopentol, iohexol and metrizoate on the contractile force of the isolated rabbit heart. Acta Radiol Suppl (Stockh) 370: 61
5. Als AV, Serur JR, LaRaia PJ, Miner N, Paulin S (1978) Differential effects of sodium meglumine calcium metrizoate on the inotropic state of normal and ischemic myocardium. Radiology 128: 499
6. Anonymous (1949) Un nuovo agente solubilizzante. It Farmaco Sci 4: 122
7. Aronson RS, Cranefield PF (1974) The effect of resting potential on the electrical activity of canine cardiac purkinje fibers exposed to Na-free solution or oubain. Pflugers Arch 347: 101
8. Bååth L (1990) Sodium addition and/or oxygen saturation of the nonionic contrast medium iohexol during normal and reduced perfusion pressure in the isolated rabbit heart. Effects on contractile force and risk of ventricular fibrillation. Acta Radiol 31: 525
9. Bååth L, Almén T (1989a) Reducing the risk of ventricular fibrillation by adding sodium to ionic and non-ionic contrast media with low iodine concentration. Coronary perfusion of the isolated rabbit heart with meglumine diatrizoate or iopentol at 140 mg I/ml and 0–154 mmol Na$^+$/l. Acta Radiol 30: 207
10. Bååth L, Almen T (1989b) Reduction of the risk of ventricular fibrillation in the isolated rabbit heart by small additions of electrolytes to nonionic monomeric contrast media. Acta Radiol 30: 327
11. Bååth L, Almén T, Öksendal A (1990) Effect of sodium addition to nonionic contrast media on cardiac contractile force. Perfusion of the isolated rabbit heart with iohexol and iopentol containing 0–154 mmol Na$^+$/l added as NaCl. Acta Radiol 31: 99
12. Bååth L, Almén T, Öksendal A (1990) Oxygen saturation of the low osmolar contrast media iohexol, ioxaglate and iodixanol in the isolated rabbit heart. Acta Radiol 31: 519
13. Bailey JC, Elharrar V, Douglas PZ (1978) Slow-channel depolarization: mechanism and control of arrhythmias. Ann Rev Med 29: 417
14. Beeler GW, Reuter H (1977) Reconstruction of the action potential of ventricular myocardial fibers. J Physiol (Lond) 268: 177
15. Blanke H, Rentrop P, Karsch KR, Kreuzer H (1979) Coronary angiographic and ventriculographic findings in the acute and chronic stage of myocardial infarction. Circulation 60 [Suppl]: 11
16. Boijsen E, Kormano M (eds) (1987) Iopentol Chemistry, toxicology and pharmacology of a non-ionic contrast medium. Acta Radiol Suppl 370
17. de Burgh Daly I, Clark AJ (1921) The action of ions upon the frog's heart. J Physiol (Lond) 54: 367
18. Bygrave FL (1978) Mitochondria and the control of intracellular calcium. Biol Rev 53: 43
19. Chapman RA (1983) Control of cardiac contractility at the cellular level. Am J Physiol 245: H535
20. Cranefield PF, Wit AL, Hoffman BF (1972) Conduction of the cardiac impulse. III. Characteristics of very slow conduction. J Gen Physiol 59: 227
21. Davis K, Ward Kennedy J, Kemp HG Jr, Judkins MP, Gosselin AJ, Killip T (1979) Complications of coronary arteriography from the collaborative study of coronary artery surgery (CASS). Circulation 59: 1105
22. Dawson P, Bradshaw A (1989) Radiocontrast agents are contact activators of coagulation. Br J Radiol 62: 631
23. Dawson P, Howell M (1986) The nonionic dimers: a new class of contrast agents. Br J Radiol 59: 987
24. Dhalla NS, Smith CI, Pierce GN, Elimban V, Makino N, Khattar JC (1986) Heart sarcolemmal cation pumps and binding sites. *In:* Rupp H (ed) Regulation of heart function: basic concepts and clinical applications. Thieme, New York, p 121
25. Dhalla NS, Ziegelhoffer A, Harrow JAC (1977) Regulatory role of membrane systems in heart function. Can J Physiol Pharmacol 55: 1211
26. Fabiato A (1983) Calcium-induced release of calcium from the cardiac sarcoplasmatic reticulum. Am J Physiol 245: C1
27. Fabiato A, Fabiato F (1977) Calcium release from the sarcoplasmatic reticulum. Circ Res 40: 119
28. Feinberg H, Boyd E, Tanzini G (1968) Mechanical performance and oxygen utilization of the isolvolumic rabbit heart. Am J Physiol 215: 132
29. Feldman RL, Jalowiec DA, Hill JA, Lambert CR (1988) Contrast media-related complications during cardiac catheterization using Hexabrix or Renografin in high-risk patients. Am J Cardiol 61: 1334
30. Fischer HW (1986) Catalogue of intravascular contrast media. Radiology 159: 561
31. Fischer HW, Thomson KR (1978) Contrast media in coronary arteriograhy: a review. Invest Radiol 13: 450
32. Garrey WE (1914) The nature of fibrillatory contractions. Its relation to tissue mass and form. Am. J. Physiol 33: 397
33. Gerber KH, Higgins CB, Yuh Y, Koziol JA (1982) Regional myocardial hemodynamic and metabolic effects of ionic and nonionic contrast media in normal and ischemic states. Circulation 65: 1307

34. Gertz EW, Wisneski JA, Neese R, Silverstein D, Akin JR, Morris DL (1984) The effects of iopamidol on myocardial metabolism. A comparison with Renografin-76. Invest Radiol [Suppl] 19: S191.
35. Gillum RF (1987) Coronary bypass surgery and coronary angiography in the United States, 1979–1983. Am Heart J 113: 1255
36. Grainger RG (1980) Osmolality of intravascular radiological contrast media. Br J Radiol 53: 739
37. Hayakawa K, Yamashita K (1989) Low-osmolality contrast media-induced ventricular fibrillation. Invest Radiol 24: 298
38. Hesselink JR, Hayman LA, Chung KJ, McGinnis BD, Davis KR Taveras JM (1984) Myocardial ischemia during intravenous DSA in patients with cardiac disease. Radiology 153: 577
39. Higgins CB (1984a) Overview of cardiovascular effects of contrast media. Comparison of ionic and non-ionic media. Invest Radiol [Suppl] 19: S187
40. Higgins CB (1984b) Contrast media in the cardiovascular system. *In*: Sovak M (ed) Radiocontrast agents. Springer, Berlin Heidelberg New York, p 193 (Handbook of experimental pharmacology, vol 73)
41. Hohenjäger P (1986) Regulation of myocardial force of contractile by sarcolemmal ion channels, the sodium pump, and sodium-calcium exchange. *In*: Rupp H (ed) Regulation of heart function: basic concepts and clinical applications. Thieme New York p 159
42. Katayama H, Yamaguchi K, Kozuka T, Takashima T, Seez P, Matsuura K (1990) Adverse reactions to ionic and nonionic contrast media. A report from the Japanese committee on the safety of contrast media. Radiology 175: 621
43. Katz AM (1977) Cardiac action potential. *In*: Katz AM (ed) Physiology of the heart. Raven, New York, 229.
44. Kinnison ML, Powe NR, Steinberg EP (1989) Results of randomized controlled trials of low-versus high-osmolality contrast media. Radiology 170: 381
45. Kohlhart M, Haastert HP, Krause H (1973) Evidence of non-specificity of the Ca-channel in mammalian myocardial fibre membranes. Pflugers Arch 342: 125
46. Kozeny GA, Murdock DK, Euler DE, Hano JE, Scanlon PJ, Bansal VK, Vertuno LL (1984) In vivo effects of acute changes in osmolality and sodium concentration on myocardial contractility. Am Heart J 109: 290
47. Langendorff O (1895) Untersuchangen am überlebenden Säugetierherzen. Pflugers Arch Ges Physiol 61: 219
48. Langer GA (1971) The intrinsic control of myocardial contraction – ionic factors. N Engl J Med 285: 1065
49. Langer GA (1987) The role of calcium at the sarcolemma in the control of myocardial contractility. Can J Physiol Pharmacol 65: 627
50. Langer GA, Frank JS, Philipson KD (1982) Ultrastructure and calcium exchange of the sarcolemma, sarcoplasmatic reticulum and mitochondria of the myocardium. Pharmacol Ther 16: 331
51. Lasser EC, Berry CC (1989) Nonionic vs ionic contrast media: what do the data tell us? Am J Roentgenol 152: 985
52. Lee CO (1981) Ionic activities in cardiac muscle cell and application of ion-selective microelectrodes. Am J Physiol 241: H459
53. Lee CO (1985) 200 years of digitalis: the emerging central role of sodium in the control of cardiac force. Am J Physiol 249: C367
54. Lee CO, Fozzard HA (1975) Activities of potassium and sodium ions in rabbit heart muscle. J Gen Physiol 65: 695
55. McAllister RE, Noble D, Tsien RW (1975) Reconstruction of the action potential of cardiac purkinje firbers. J Physiol (Lond) 251: 1
56. McAlpin RN, Weidner WA, Kattus AA, Hanafee WN (1966) Electrocardiographic changes during selective coronary cineangiograhy. Circulation 34: 627
57. McEwen LM (1956) The effect on the isolated rabbit heart of vagal stimulation and its modification by cocaine, hexamethonium and oubain. J Physiol (Lond) 131: 678
58. Miller D, Lohse J, Wolf GL (1976) Slow response in canine purkinje fiber by contrast medium. Invest Radiol 11: 577
59. Mines GR (1914) On circulating excitations in the heart muscle and their possible relation to tachycardia and fibrillation. Trans R Soc Can 8: 43
60. Morgan HE, James RN (1985) Metobolic regulation and myocardial function. *In*: Willis Hurst J (ed) The heart, 6th ed; MacGraw-Hill, New York, p 16
61. Morris TW (1988) The importance of sodium concentration on the incidence of fibrillation during coronary arteriography in dogs. Invest Radiol [Suppl] 23: 137
62. Morris TW, Ventura J (1986) Incidence of fibrillation with dilute contrast media for intra-arterial coronary digital substracted angiography. Invest Radiol 21: 416

63. Morris TW, Hayakawa K, Sahler LG, Ekholm S (1986) Incidence of fibrillation with isotonic contrast media for intra-arterial coronary digital subtraction angiography. Diagn Imag Clin Med 55: 109
64. Mullins LJ (1979) The generation of electric currents in cardiac fibers by Na/Ca exchange. Am J Physiol 236: C103
65. Murdock DK, Euler DE, Becker DM, Murdock JD, Scanlon PJ, Gunnar RM (1985) Ventricular fibrillation during coronary angiography: an analysis of mechanisms. Am Heart J 109: 265
66. Neagley SR, Vought MB, Weidner WA, Zwillich CW (1986) Transient oxygen desaturation following radiographic contrast medium administration. Arch Intern Med 146: 1094
67. Neely JR, Liebermeister H, Battersby EJ, Morgan HE (1967) Effect of pressure development on oxygen consumption by isolated rat heart. Am J Physiol 212: 804
68. New W, Trautwein W (1972) Inward membrane currents in mammalian myocardium. Pflugers Arch 334: 1
69. Newell JD, Higgins CB, Kelley MJ, Green CF, Schmidt WS Haigler F (1980) The influence of hyperosmolality on left ventricular contractile state: disparate effects of nonionic and ionic solutions. Invest Radiol 15: 363
70. Paulin S, Adams DF (1971) Increased ventricular fibrillation during coronary arteriography with a new contrast medium preparation. Radiology 101: 45
71. Reeves J, Trumble W, Sutko JL, Kadoma M, Fröhlich J (1981) Calcium transport mechanisms in cardiac sarcolemmal vesicles. In: Bronner F, Peterlik M (eds) Calcium and phosphate transport across biomembranes. Academic, New York, p 15
72. Reuter H, Seitz N (1968) The dependence of calcium efflux from cardiac muscle on temperature and external ion composition. J Physiol (Lond) 195: 451
73. Russell DC, Oliver MF (1978) Ventricular refractoriness during acute myocardial ischaemia and its relationship to ventricular fibrillation. Cardiovasc Res 12: 221
74. Rüegg JC, Pfitzer G (1986) Excitation-contraction coupling in coronary smooth muscle. In: Rupp H (ed) Regulation of heart function: basic concepts and clinical applications. Thieme, New York, p 22
75. Salvesen S, Lund Nielsen P, Holtermann H (1967) Ameliorating effects of calcium and magnesium ions on the toxicity of isopaque sodium. II: Studies on the isolated heart and auricles of the rabbit. Acta Radiol Suppl 270: 17
76. Serur JR, Als AV, Miner-Green N, Paulin S (1980) Comparative effects of three radiographic contrast agents in isolated normal and ischemic canine hearts. Invest Radiol 15: 196
77. Silver PJ (1986) Pharmacological modulation of cardiac and vascular contractile protein function. J Cardiovasc Pharmacol 8 [Suppl 9]: 34
78. Simon AL, Shabetai R, Lang JH, Lasser EC (1972) The mechanism of production of ventricular fibrillation in coronary angiography. Am J Roentgenol 114: 810
79. Sovak M, Robertson HJ (1988) Osmolality and ionicity: confusion in terminology applied to contrast media (letter). Radiology 168: 281
80. Starling EH (1918) The Linacre lecture on the law of the heart. Longman, Green & O., London
81. Surawicz B (1967) Relationship between electrocardiogram and electrolytes. Am Heart J 73: 814
82. Swick M (1929) Darstellung der Niere und Harnwege in Röntgenbild durch intravenöse Einbringung eines neuen Kontraststoffes: des Uroselectans. Klin Wochenschr 8: 2087
83. Thomson KR, Violante MR, Kenyon T, Fischer HW (1978) Reduction of ventricular fibrillation using calcium-enriched Renografin 76. Invest Radiol 13: 238
84. Tilly P, Hardouin M, Lautrou J (1974) Kontrastmittel für Röntgenaufnahmen. Bundesrepublik Deutschland, Offenlegungsschrift 2523567
85. Trägårdh B, Lynch PR (1987) Cardiac effects of ionic and nonionic contrast agents. In: Parvez Z, Moncada R, Sovak M (eds) Contrast media: biologic effects and clinical application, vol 2. CRC, Boca Raton
86. Trägårdh B, Almén T, Lynch P (1975) Addition of calcium or other cations and of oxygen to ionic and nonionic contrast media. Effects on cardiac function during coronary arteriography. Invest Radiol 10: 231
87. Tsien RW (1983) Calcium channels in excitable membranes. Ann Rev Physiol 45: 341
88. Vik-Mo H, Rosland G, Fölling M, Danielsen R (1988) Hemodynamic and electrocardiographic consequenses of high- and low-osmolality contrast agents for left ventricular angiography. Cathet Cardiovasc Diagn 14: 143
89. Ward Kennedy J, Baxley WA, Bunnel IL, Gensini GG, Messer JV, Mudd JG, Noto TJ, Paulin S, Pichard AD, Sheldon WC, Cohen M (1982) Mortality related to cardiac catheterization and mortality. Cathet Cardiovasc Diagn 8: 323
90. Weikl A, Drust OE, Lang E (1975) Komplikationen der selektiven Koronarangiographie in Abhängigkeit von verwendeten Kontrastmitteln. ROFO 123: 218

91. Weirich J, Antoni H (1986) Vulnerability of the heart to ventricular fibrillation: basic mechanisms. *In:* Rupp H (ed) Regulation of heart function. Thieme New York, p 376
92. Weisfeldt ML, Shock NW (1970) Effect of perfusion pressure on coronary flow and oxygen usage of nonworking heart. Am J Physiol 218: 95
93. Wit AL, Rosen MR, Hoffman BF (1974) Electrophysiology and pharmacology of cardiac arrhythmias. II. Relationship of normal and abnormal electrical activity of cardiac fibers to the genesis of arrhythmias. Am Heart J 88: 515
94. Wolf GL (1980) The fibrillatory properties of contrast agents. Invest Radiol 15: 208
95. Wolf GL, Mulry CS, Laski PA, Kilzer K (1983) Changes in ventricular fibrillation threshold induced by contrast agents during acute coronary artery occlusion. Invest Radiol 18: 145
96. Yamazaki H, Banka VS, Bodenheimer MM, Hattori S, Agarwal JB, Helfant RH (1980) Differential effects of Renografin-76 in the ischemic and monischemic myocardium. Am J Cardiol 47: 597

Clinical Magnetic Resonance Spectroscopy—The Present State

O. Henriksen and K.E. Jensen

1 Introduction

Through the last decade magnetic resonance imaging (MRI) has developed into a powerful, and by now well established, diagnostic imaging modality. The clinical use of magnetic resonance spectroscopy (MRS) has, however, shown a rather slow rate of progression. This may be explained partly by the extensive technical requirements of human in vivo MRS, such as: quality of tissue volume selection, acceptable magnetic field homogeneity (shimming), and sufficiently skilled technologists and physicians. Furthermore, low in vivo concentrations of the metabolites of interest together with the inherent low sensitivity (low signal-to-noise

Danish Research Center of Magnetic Resonance, Hvidovre Hospital, University of Copenhagen, DK-2650 Copenhagen, Denmark

Frontiers in European Radiology, Vol. 8
Eds. Baert/Heuck
© Springer-Verlag, Berlin Heidelberg 1991

ratio) of the MRS experiment provide extreme difficulties for the implementation of MRS as a clinical modality. It is obvious, however, that MRS of humans is the only technique in clinical medicine that provides noninvasive insight to tissue biochemistry in vivo, and thus offers a substantial research potential. The use of MRS as a clinical diagnostic modality has, despite a growing amount of knowledge during the last 5 years, yet to prove its efficacy.

The aim of the present review is to provide critical assessment of the future clinical potential in the light of the very latest research results from patients [18, 21, 66, 86,112].

2 Technical Aspects

To get a proper understanding of the diagnostic value spectroscopy may provide in clinical practice it is important to review the methods most frequently used in human in vivo studies. In MRI a general agreement on methods for spatial localization was reached only a few years after the first clinical scanners were taken into operation, but in MRS the number of methods and strategies is almost as high as the number of pathological conditions investigated. Furthermore, where the most frequently used MRI method for volume selection (two-dimensional Fourier transform) in principle is simple, the spectroscopic methods are frequently quite complex. The principal reason for this is the relatively low signal-to-noise ratio of most biochemical species caused by the low in vivo concentrations. Where a conventional diagnostic MRI signal is derived from the protons of tissue water and lipid, the signal from most metabolites of interest in MRS is a factor of 10^5 lower. The majority of clinical MRS studies up to now have used the signal from either phosphorus (^{31}P) or protons (^1H). In an excellent review by *Aue* [9] a large number of methods for volume selection in vivo have been described, and in the following only a brief overview of the methods most frequently used in patient studies will be given.

2.1 Simple Surface Coil Technique

The simple surface coil technique, where a surface coil serves both as radio frequency (RF) transmitter and receiver, has essentially been the first technique for human in vivo spectroscopy and is still the most important method for animal studies. The geometry and size of the surface coil define the sensitive volume from which the MRS signals derive. The surface coil technique remains the most robust technique and provides excellent measurement data when the pathological condition does not require accurate volume selection. The method has been used in the majority of clinical examinations of skeletal muscle and works well in exercise models. Two of the drawbacks of the method are the inhomogeneity in excitation (inhomogeneity in B1 field) and the very poor definition of the signal giving tissue volume.

2.2 Complex Surface Coil Techniques

A number of modifications of the simple surface coil technique have been developed in order to overcome the poor definition of the selected tissue volume. The rotating frame (RTF) method uses localizing spatial gradients in the surface coil RF excitation in order to select tissue "slices" at different distances from the surface coil. A version of the RTF method with two surface coils (a large coil for excitation and a small for signal reception) has been described by *Styles* et al. [103] and has been used for a number of patient studies.

Another surface coil technique, the topical magnetic resonance (TMR) method, uses a magnetic field gradient in the static field (main field, B0) to create field inhomogeneity except for the tissue volume of interest relative to the detecting surface coil [43]. The drawback of the TMR technique is that the selected tissue volume is still rather poorly defined and cannot be moved in position.

A third rather complex technique, proposed by *Bottomley* et al. [25], is depth-resolved surface coil spectroscopy (DRESS). This technique uses the inhomogeneous RF excitation of the surface coil together with a magnetic field gradient. The signals from a slice defined by the gradient and the sensitive volume of the surface coil are detected. One advantage of the DRESS technique is that it permits signal detection from several slices at different distances from the surface coil. The occurrence of eddy currents due to the gradient switching interferes with the signal detection and remains a drawback of the technique.

2.3 Image-Selected In Vivo Spectroscopy

In image-selected in vivo spectroscopy (ISIS) originally proposed by *Ordidge* et al. [81], pulsed orthogonal magnetic field gradients together with selective 180° RF pulses are used. A cubic tissue volume can be selected as a result of addition/subtraction of eight experiments. The major advantage of the ISIS technique as compared to the surface coil methods described above is the fact that the tissue volume of interest (VOI) can be selected from a standard MRI image and the positioning performed without moving the patient. Furthermore, the ISIS technique utilizes the same physical methods as MRI and thus permits a high degree of clinical feasibility for patient examinations in connection with MRI. One drawback of the ISIS technique is, however, that selection of relatively small volumes (below $3 \times 3 \times 3 \, cm^3$) is associated with difficulties caused by the signal addition/subtraction inherent to the ISIS technique (i.e., subtraction of large signals to give the very small signal from the tissue VOI), but this can partly be overcome by incorporation of a surface coil (improvement of signal-to-noise ratio) for MR-signal reception.

2.4 Stimulated Echo Acquisition Mode

In stimulated echo acquisition mode (STEAM) [40, 41] three slice-selective 90° RF pulses applied in the presence of three consecutive orthogonal magnetic field gradients are used. This method creates a signal (stimulated echo) from a cubic VOI within a single experiment, and the position and size of the VOI is defined by the frequency and bandwidth of the selective 90° RF pulses. A major advantage of this technique is that it permits selective T1 and T2 relaxation time measurements within a selected tissue volume. Another feature of the STEAM technique is that it permits genuine solvent suppressed spectroscopy from patients, which is extremely important for proton spectroscopy since many important metabolites are obscured by the large resonance from tissue water protons. Thus, it is only possible after a water-suppressed RF pulse before the actual STEAM experiment to detect tissue metabolites with low concentration in vivo (i.e., lactate). The STEAM technique has only been implemented very recently on clinical MR scanners but has already proved to be an excellent technique for clinical proton spectroscopy.

2.5 Spatially Resolved Spectroscopy

In spatially resolved spectroscopy (SPARS) presented by *Luyten* et al. [70], selective RF pulses (both 90° and 180°) in the presence of magnetic field gradients are used to select a tissue VOI. The size of the selected VOI can be altered by changing the bandwidth of the selective RF pulse or by changing the gradient field strength used. The method also permits the acquisition of signals from a selected tissue VOI within a single experiment.

One disadvantage of the SPARS technique is the limited possibility for in vivo water-suppressed MRS which generally results in low spectral quality. This technique also provides the possibility for selective relaxation time measurements in the VOI because SPARS can be combined with classical inversion recovery and multiple spin echo pulse sequences [69].

2.6 Chemical Shift Imaging

Several methods have been proposed for use of the chemical shift phenomenon to improve the diagnostic potential of MRI or acquire chemical information from living tissues. The theory and principles of chemical shift imaging (CSI) methods have previously been reviewed [29, 30]. The methods most frequently used for patient investigations so far (proton methods) are the chemical shift selective imaging (CHESS) method proposed by *Frahm* et al. [42], the modified spin echo method proposed by *Dixon* [38], and the inversion-recovery method with short inversion time (STIR).

The CHESS method uses an RF pulse to suppress the MR signal from tissue water protons or lipid protons, respectively, in order to create "water" and "fat" images by subtraction. This method has proven useful for studies of a variety of pathological conditions in patients, involving quantitative changes in fat to water ratio of the tissue of interest. The Dixon method uses the difference in nuclear precession rate (difference in phase) between the protons in tissue water and lipids and creates images that are dependent on either the water or fat content of the tissue.

Preliminary clinical results have been reported regarding CSI methods for imaging of phosphorus [23, 110, 117]. The major problem for the phosphorus CSI methods is the very short T2 relaxation times of phosphorus metabolites [108]. The inherent low signal-to-noise ratio (in four-dimensional CSI) provides a poor spatial resolution, and the computation demands in four-dimensional CSI are still rather fierce since the two-dimensional "metabolic image" is created from a four-dimensional Fourier transformed data set. Thus, automatization of signal processing in phosphorus CSI seems mandatory.

3 Processing and Evaluation of Spectroscopy Data

The first quantitative method for evaluating *in vivo* human spectroscopic results was measurement of resonance (peak) height or area. The parameters are compared to each other resulting in peak ratios (i.e., phosphocreatine to inorganic phosphate ratio). These ratios are chosen on the basis of their biochemical relevance in the given spectroscopic study (i.e., comparison of phosphorus spectra from skeletal muscle before and during exercise, comparison between tumor spectra and spectra from normal tissue). The peak areas can also be related to the sum of all the peak areas in the spectrum—the total MR signal. This method provides a number of advantages: instrument (hardware) changes and other systematic factors are eliminated, but the major drawback is the lack of definite actual metabolite concentrations. There is a growing need to obtain absolute metabolite concentrations from spectroscopic data, but so far no reliable method has emerged for clinical use. Only very preliminary results have reported actual metabolite concentrations from clinical examinations of humans. These methods have either used tissue extracts or internal standard (i.e., water concentration), but the reliability and precision have to be proved.

Another factor of major importance is the postprocessing of the spectroscopic measurements. The postprocessing includes multiplication, filtering, phase correction, and sometimes additional baseline correction. The variation in postprocessing routine together with the frequent lack of detailed description in published results provide a major limitation for comparison of spectroscopic data obtained on different MR scanners. Accurate quality control studies of methods for postprocessing of spectroscopic data and integration of peak areas are requested in order to secure comparable, reliable and precise clinical results.

4 Skeletal Muscle

4.1 Phosphorus Sectroscropy

Since the late 1970s the interest in MRS of muscles has grown rapidly because of its noninvasive nature. ^{31}P-MRS provides the possibility for direct examination of muscle bioenergetics since ATP, phosphocreatine (PCr), and inorganic phosphate (Pi) are readily resolved in clinical phosphorus spectra. Since the chemical shift of Pi relative to PCr is pH sensitive, ^{31}P-MRS provides pH measurements from the muscle tissue during stress (i.e., exercise). The number of possible exercise models for human studies is limited due to the design of the MR scanners and has so far been proposed for the flexor muscles of the hand [87] and for the calf muscles [114, 85]. The majority of clinical studies have investigated ischemic disorders and inborn errors of muscle metabolism which affect high-energy phosphate metabolism (enzyme deficiencies).

Of the inborn errors, McArdle's syndrome is perhaps the best investigated, and 15 patients have been investigated with ^{31}P-MRS and reported in the literature [55]. In McArdle's syndrome there is a lack of activation of the enzyme glycogen phosphorylase which regulates the degradation of glycogen. Thus, no lactic acid is produced during muscle exercise and PCr is degraded at a faster rate than in normal skeletal muscle. In ^{31}P-MRS these processes result in excessive reductions in the PCr resonance, as seen in Fig. 1, and absence of the expected pH reduction [3, 55]. The major advantage of ^{31}P-MRS in the investigation of inborn errors of muscle metabolism is the noninvasive nature of the method, which provides the possibility for limitless numbers of repeated examinations. Thus, it is possible to use ^{31}P-MRS to monitor eventual changes and effects of therapy, as demonstrated in McArdle's syndrome where attempts to substitute muscle glycogen consumption for energy expenditure have been evaluated with ^{31}P-MRS during exercise [3, 55].

A large number of clinical studies of patients with inborn errors of muscle metabolism have been conducted so far. The majority of reports of such patients have been published by *Radda* and coworkers [87, 46, 104] and *Chance* and

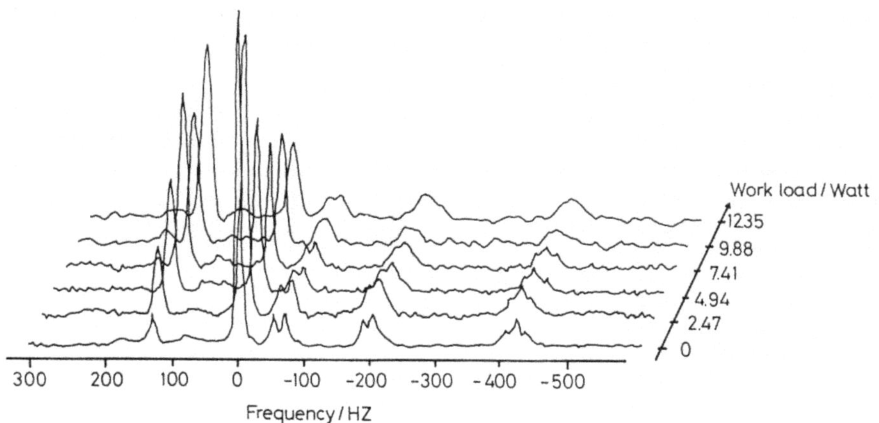

Fig. 1. Stacked plot of ^{31}P-spectra obtained before and during different levels of work load in a McArdle patient. Five resonances can be identified from left to right: Pi, PCr, γ-ATP, α-ATP, and β-ATP. Note the decrease in PCr and the corresponding increase in Pi during exercise. (From [55])

coworkers [4–6, 34]. Furthermore, extensive research in normal muscle exercise physiology has been conducted and a broad knowledge base of basic muscle energetics has been brought forward which serve as a reference for current investigations [10, 19, 75, 74, 105].

Clinical investigations of ischemic disorders such as peripheral arterial occlusive disease have been few [44, 61, 114], but have emphasized the potential for ^{31}P-MRS in evaluating the tissue perfusion. All studies found a prolonged recovery rate after exercise in patients with arterial occlusive disease of the lower extremities. Phosphocreatine was, furthermore, used at a faster rate in patients with occlusive arterial disease than in normal subjects. None of these studies could detect any abnormalities in ^{31}P spectra from the muscle tissue of the patients during rest, which emphasizes the importance of an exercise model (ergometer) and a thoroughly evaluated control group. The diagnostic value of ^{31}P-MRS in patients suffering from occlusive arterial disease has to be compared with the simple and inexpensive physiological methods using strain gauge techniques for measurements of peripheral arterial pressure.

In patients suffering from Duchenne's muscular dystrophy ^{31}P spectra have, however, shown abnormal Pi to PCr ratios [12] which suggests a potential for ^{31}P-MRS in the evaluation of patients with neuromuscular disorders.

^{31}P-MRS of skeletal muscle may be useful in the study of suffering from unspecific weakness, fatigue, and muscle pain. Abnormal muscle energetics have been observed in postviral exhaustion syndrome [8], unspecific muscle pain [104], and primary fibromyalgia [59]. Research in these very frequent but poorly characterized muscle disorders may benefit from ^{31}P-MRS investigation with respect to further clarification of the pathogenesis and possible evaluation of therapy [62]. Abnormal phosphorus energetics have been reported in skeletal muscle during exercise in patients with congestive heart failure [90, 71, 113]. The phosphocreatine utilization and decrease in intracellular pH during exercise is significantly greater in patients suffering from congestive heart failure than in normal controls. These observations could prove to be of major importance to the investigation of peripheral muscular response to cardiac disorders.

4.2 Proton Spectroscopy

So far only a limited number of proton spectroscopic studies have been reported. *Narayana* et al. [77] have investigated the gastrocnemius muscles in 12 normal volunteers and report very little interindividual change in the water resonance, but substantial variation in the region of the lipid resonances. *Barany* et al. [11] have also examined the gastrocnemius muscles in normal subjects but have compared the results with patients suffering from primary or secondary muscular disorders (i.e., Duchenne's dystrophy, myotonic dystrophy, Charcot–Marie–Tooth disease, cerebral palsy, Werdnig–Hoffmann disease, and spina bifida). A number of variations in the region of the lipid resonances are reported [14, 78], but the number of patients is still limited, so the clinical value remains unclear at the present time.

5 Brain

The majority of clinical spectroscopic investigations of the brain have so far dealt with: intracranial tumors, vascular disorders, white matter lesions, and metabolic conditions (i.e., coma caused by liver disease); but studies of normal brain metabolism have been conducted in order to characterize regional differences [26] and metabolic state during varying physiological conditions [59, 111].

5.1 Intracranial Tumors

Figure 2 shows an axial T_2-weighted MR image from a patient with a cerebral tumor (astrocytoma, grade grade III) in the right cerebral hemisphere.

Figure 3a shows a phosphorus spectrum (at 1.5 T) obtained with the ISIS technique from normal brain tissue in the left cerebral hemisphere (the VOI is $5 \times 5 \times 5 \, cm^3$). A total of seven phosphorus resonances can be resolved (from left to right): phosphomonoesters (PME), Pi, phosphodiesters (PDE), PCr, and γ-, α-, β-ATP.

Phosphorus spectroscopy of large superficial brain tumors using simple surface coil techniques has been among the first clinical investigations performed on clinically operating MR scanners. Only subtle differences have been observed between tumor spectra and spectra from normal brain tissue [94, 107]. Even large highly malignant brain tumors with substantial tissue necroses have shown normal phosphorus spectra and only marginal deviations in pH values. A possible explanation for these findings may be that a substantial amount of the signals from adjacent normal neuronal tissue have been included in the recorded spectra

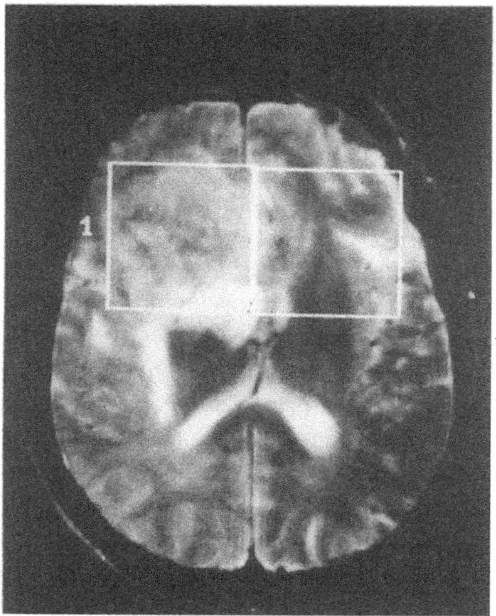

Fig. 2. An axial T2-weighted MR image from a patient with a large astrocytoma (grade III) in the right frontal cerebral hemisphere. One cubic VOI $(5 \times 5 \times 5 \, cm^3)$ has been selected in the left normal cerebral hemisphere and another VOI $(5 \times 5 \times 5 \, cm^3)$ has been selected within the tumor (1) in the right cerebral hemisphere

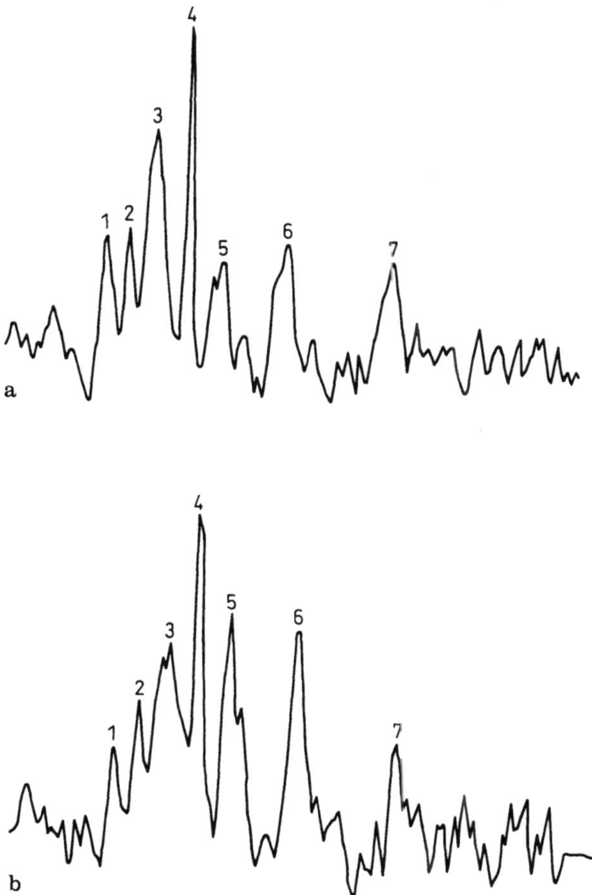

Fig. 3a, b. A-three-dimensional phosphorus spectrum **a** from the cubic VOI of *normal brain* shown in Fig. 2, and **b** from the VOI selected within the tumor shown in Fig. 2. The resonances of (from left to right) phosphomonoesters (*1*), inorganic phosphate (*2*), phosphodiesters (*3*), phosphocreatine (*4*), γ-ATP (*5*), α-ATP (*6*), and β-ATP (*7*) could be identified. Both spectra were acquired with the ISIS technique and no differences could be seen in the spectrum from the tumor compared with the contralateral normal brain spectrum

by the simple surface coil technique (crude localization). However, spectroscopic investigations performed with improved precision in volume selection (ISIS technique) have generally given similar results [97, 98]; an example is seen in Fig. 3b. An increase in the relative concentration of PMEs has been observed in some of the tumors [97]. Furthermore, changes have been observed in spectra from tumors in relation to treatment with radiation therapy [97]. At the present stage in technological development no clear conclusions can be drawn from the ^{31}P-spectroscopic investigations of intracranial tumors in humans. In comparison with high-resolution MRI, no additional new diagnostic information can be derived from phosphorus spectra from intracranial tumors in humans, but improved technical methods (capable of selection of small volumes $< 1\,\text{cm}^3$) may reduce the partial volume problem. Quantification of absolute concentrations may well provide important new data and improve the sensitivity of ^{31}P-spectroscopic examinations of human brain tumors [52, 53]. Another significant problem is the lack of studies investigating precision and quality of the volume-selective methods used in the clinical patient studies, since investigations on a standard reference test phantom, provided by the EEC Concerted Action on tissue characterization, have indicated that up to 30% of the detected MR signal (ISIS technique) may originate from outside the selected volume.

Methods using localized water suppressed proton spectroscopy indicate that additional diagnostic information may be obtained from intracranial tumors, and that tissue characterization (noninvasive "biopsy") may in fact be a future possibility [31, 49]. An example of a water-suppressed proton spectrum (at 1.5 T) obtained with the STEAM technique from the left brain hemisphere $(4 \times 4 \times 4\,\text{cm}^3)$ of a normal volunteer (shown in Fig. 4) is given with the chemical shift of the detectable metabolites in Fig. 5. Five metabolites can be resolved (from left to right): inositols, taurine, cholines (CHO), creatine/phosphocreatine (CR/PCr) and N-acetyl aspartate (NAA).

Generally, a relative decrease in NAA is seen in water-suppressed spectra from intracranial brain tumors together with a concomitant increase in CHO [31, 48]. In intracranial tumors with tissue necroses the resonance of lactate can be resolved (as seen in Fig. 7). Spectral differences characteristic of "malignant" lesions have been indicated by *Bruhn* et al. [31], primarily involving occurrence of the lactate resonance which is not present in brain tissue during normal physiological conditions. However, the clinical relevance of proton spectroscopy of intracranial tumors is not clarified at present and further research must be carried out in order to clarify: absolute quantification of metabolite concentrations, evaluation of

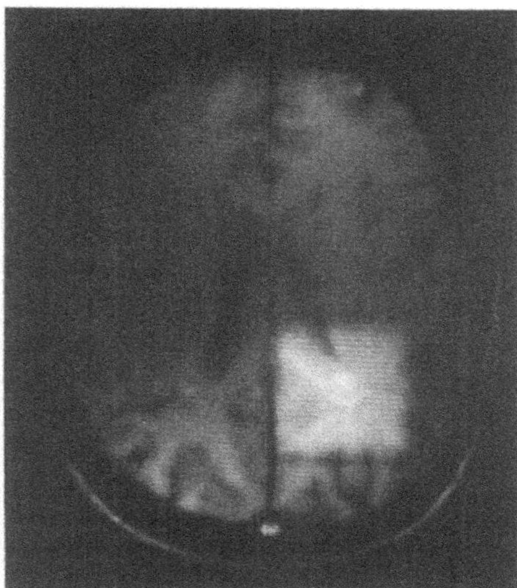

Fig. 4. Axial fast low angle shot (FLASH) MR image of the brain in a normal volunteer. The VOI $(4 \times 4 \times 4\,\text{cm}^3)$ selected for localized water-suppressed proton spectroscopy is super-imposed. (From [48])

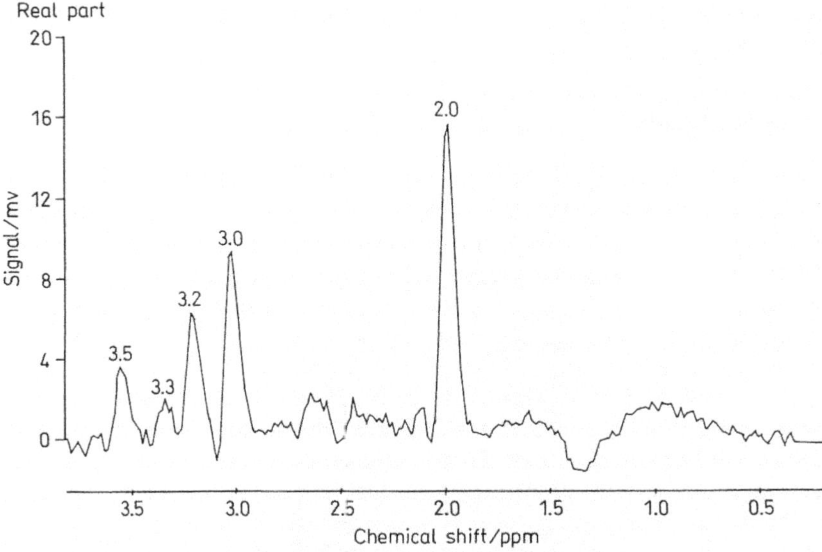

Fig. 5. Water-suppressed proton spectrum from the cubic VOI in the normal brain shown in Fig. 4. The resonances were assigned as follows: inositols (3.5 ppm), taurine (3.3 pmm), cholines (3.2 ppm), creatine/phosphocreatine (3.0 ppm), and NAA (2.0 ppm). (From [48])

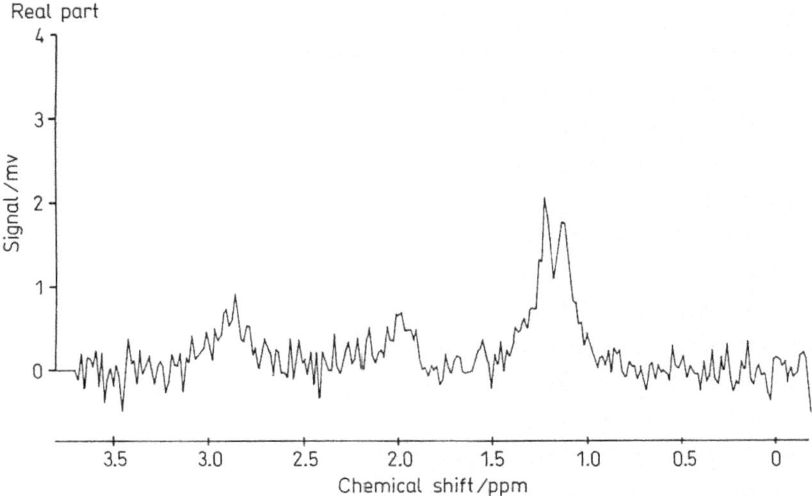

Fig. 6. Water-suppressed proton spectrum obtained with the STEAM technique from a VOI ($4 \times 4 \times 4\,cm^3$) within a large cerebral infarct. The spectrum is dominated by a large lactate resonance, whereas the "normal" metabolities (NAA, creatine/phosphocreatine, choline) are hardly detectable. (From [48])

regional variations within the tumors [99], and methodological precision of the spectral acquisition.

5.2 Vascular Disorders

Stroke patients have been studied with phosphorus spectroscopy as well as with water-suppressed proton spectroscopy. Serial studies (using the TMR technique) indicate a reduction in PCr to Pi ratio during the first 7 days after the insult [67]. In chronic cerebral infraction there seems to be a general reduction in all phosphorus metabolites [24, 79, 67]. Water-suppressed proton spectroscopy has shown marked metabolic changes following acute stroke [32, 16, 48] within the first 3 to 4 days after the onset of symptoms. An example of a water-suppressed proton spectrum from a VOI within a large cerebral infarct is seen in Fig. 6. The proton spectrum from brain infarct is dominated by the lactate resonance, and an almost total loss of NAA, CR, and CHO. The temporal evolution remains unclear at present and systematic serial intraindividual investigations seem mandatory. One of the major experimental problems is the definition of the tissue volume within the infarct, since the delineation of infarcts by MRI remains difficult during the early time period. Regional differences within the infarct lesion, as mentioned previously, may hamper the physiological interpretation of the spectroscopic data. Nevertheless, it seems that proton spectroscopy may give valuable information

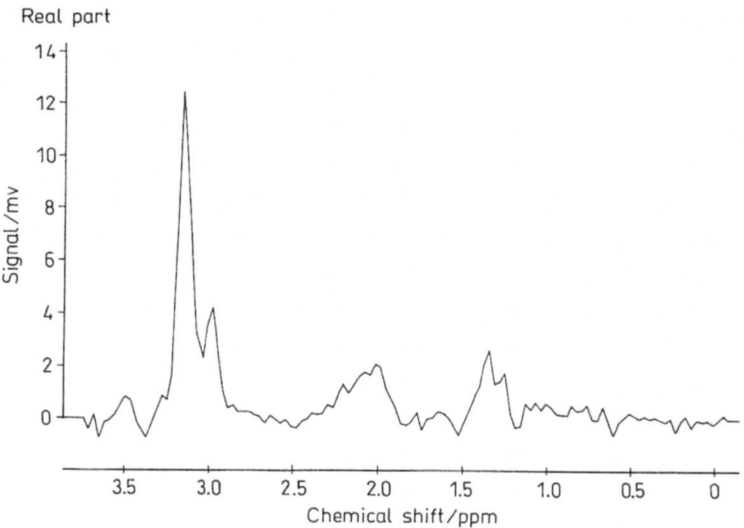

Fig. 7. A water-suppressed localized proton spectrum obtained with the STEAM technique from a VOI ($4 \times 4 \times 4\,cm^3$) within a large cerebral astrocytoma. The spectrum is dominated by a large choline resonance and a resonance with a chemical shift of 1.3 ppm corresponding to lactate. (From [48])

about the metabolic changes following acute stroke, and measurements of NAA may provide an index of neuronal cell damage.

5.3 Cerebral Hypoxia

Cerebral hypoxia due to asphyxia has been studied with phosphorus spectroscopy in newborn infants [33, 50] and may supplement blood/gas analyses and regional cerbral blood flow measurement during neonatal treatment. *Hope* and *Reynolds* [51] have reported a correlation between PCr to Pi ratios and the clinical condition in newborn infants indicating possibilities for important prognostic information in this patient group.

5.4 White Matter Lesions—Multiple Sclerosis

Only preliminary spectroscopic in vivo studies of white matter lesions (plaques) in patients with multiple sclerosis have been reported so far [7, 63]. *Arnold* et al. [7] observed a reduction in NAA to creatine ratio in chronic plaques by use of water-suppressed proton spectroscopy. In a very recent study *Larsson* et al. [63] report serial intraindividual examinations of acute plaques in order to further characterize the temporal evolution of the metabolic events that underlay the formation of the plaques. They observe a progressive decrease in the NAA to CHO ratio in acute plaques with time. An interesting finding is the appearance of lipid resonances about 2 months after the initial acute attack indicating that active demyelinization with formation of mobile fatty acids is taking place [63]. Other white matter disorders including hereditary myelin disorders and Binswanger's disease have been studied by phosphorus and proton spectroscopy. These preliminary results indicate a reduction in PDE to PCr ratio in the white matter lesions from patients with hereditary myelin disorders (detected with phosphorus spectroscopy) whereas the relative content of NAA (detected with proton spectroscopy) seems to be reduced in Binswanger's disease [68]. The results are based on a very small number of patients and do not allow any conclusions to be drawn about the underlying metabolic processes.

5.5 Metabolic Disorders

Acute hepatic encephalopathy is a condition very similar to ammonia intoxication. In patients with chronic hepatic encephalopathy a reduced Pi to ATP ratio has been reported from studies with phosphorus spectroscopy [94]. They propose a hypothesis of a "toxin" capable of inhibiting the transport of Pi into the neurons. Further investigation using localized water suppressed proton spectroscopy may clarify this hypothesis by providing data of the expected increase in intracellular glutamate/glutamine content. So far the signal-to-noise ratio has been too low to allow quantification of glutamate/glutamine resonances in brain spectra from humans.

6 Heart

Noninvasive techniques for assessing cardiac performance by evaluating the high-energy phosphorus metabolism offers unique possibilities for the investigation of ischemic heart disease. A growing number of studies have reported high-quality spectroscopic investigations of experimental models (i.e., ischemia) in animals [83, 89, 95], but very few reports have been published on heart spectroscopy in humans [22, 17]. The explanation for this discrepancy is the extreme difficulty for well-defined selection of tissue volumes inside the myocardium. Only two groups have so far been able to produce phosphorus spectra with acceptable quality. By use of the DRESS technique, a significant reduction in PCr to Pi ratio in patients with myocardial infarction, together with an elevation of the Pi to ATP ratio, have been observed [27, 28]. A study of patients with cardiomyopathy, using the RTF technique, indicates an increase in PME or PDE together with a reduced PCr/Pi ratio [88]. Phosphorus spectroscopy of the human heart in vivo is associated with great technical difficulties as the signals from the blood in the heart chambers may contribute to the MR signal because of the marginal difference in chemical shift between 2,3-diphosphoglycerate and Pi. Due to this inaccurate volume selection, phosphorus spectroscopy of the human heart seems only to be clinically feasible in patients with diffuse affection of the myocardium (i.e., enlargement as in cardiomyopathy). Technical improvements of the methods used for volume selection or application of chemical shift imaging methods may enhance the possibilities for clinical studies in the future.

7 Liver

Phosphorus spectroscopy of the liver can be performed by use of methods that avoid MR signals from the overlying muscle tissue. The phosphorus spectrum from normal liver contains only six resonances: PME, Pi, PDE, and γ-, α-, β-ATP, and hardly any PCr. In fact the lack of PCr in normal liver provides an internal "test" for the quality of the volume selection as the presence of a PCr resonance in the liver spectra indicates a signal contamination from overlying muscle [80]. Chemical shift imaging (with four-dimensional Fourier transforms) of the distribution of phosphorus metabolites has been performed in the liver [117]. As mentioned previously, these investigations require excessive use of computer power and very complex filtering algorithms and although preliminary studies have been conducted the clinical value of these methods has yet to be proven.

Phosphorus studies of patients with liver cirrhosis or steatosis have not revealed differences in the relative concentration (ratios) of high-energy phosphorus metabolites compared to normal subjects, whereas differences can be seen in liver spectra from patients with alcoholic hepatitis [2]. In a recent study of patients with alcoholic liver disease *Meyerhoff* et al. [73] tried to quantify the concentration of the phosphorus metabolites by means of the ISIS technique combined with external standards. Their report suggests a reduced concentration of phosphorus metabolites both in the patients with cirrhosis and in the patients with hepatitis, whereas there are no significant differences in the metabolite ratios. This indicates that actual quantification of the molar concentration of the observed metabolites may contribute new information, but before further clinical investigations are conducted the reliability of the quantification methods must be tested with comparative chemical analysis of liver biopsies. Thus, phosphorus spectroscopy performed without any "stress" model seems to be of limited clinical value in diffuse liver disorders. New data may be provided by use of specific functional tests in which changes in phosphorus metabolism are monitored after a metabolic stimulus. Preliminary studies have shown that it is possible to observe changes in the high-energy phosphorus metabolites in healthy subjects following an intravenous infusion of fructose [106]. In this study, a decreased Pi is observed due to increased phosphorylation of the infused fructose, resulting in an increased PME resonance [106]. Standardization of the fructose load and controlled clinical serial studies have to be performed in a larger number of normal subjects before this "stress" model can be applied in clinical use. Another "stress" model is the infusion of the amino acid alanine [36] where the phosphorylation capacity of the liver cells is tested with a stimulus similar to the fructose model. Proton CSI of the liver by use of the Dixon technique seems to be of clinical value in differentiating between focal fatty infiltration of the liver and liver metastases [47,64,65,96]. However, it does not seem possible to obtain actual quantitative measurements of liver fat content with acceptable quality using this CSI method. Localized volume selective proton spectroscopy by use of the STEAM technique seems to give a good correlation between spectroscopic data and chemically determined lipid concentration in liver biopsies (*C. Thomsen* et al., unpublished). Furthermore, preliminary results have reported abnormal proton spectra from malignant hepatic tumors [13].

8 Bone Marrow

The bone marrow offers unique possibilities for localized proton spectroscopy since it consists of the two main tissues: fat cells and hemopoietic tissue. The different composition of central hemopoietic bone marrow compared to peripheral fatty bone marrow [57] is readily seen in localized proton spectra (Fig. 8). The problem of partial volume effects present in most tissues is of minor importance in examinations of the bone marrow because of the finite location [92] within solid bone (which contributes no detectable MR signal due to the very short relaxation times). Another feature of bone marrow is that most diffuse infiltrative pathology tends to alter the tissue architecture with a major decrease in fat content. This decrease in fat tissue has been observed by localized proton spectroscopy of the tibial (fatty) bone marrow in four patients with leukemia [54]. These results have been confirmed by use of CSI methods [93,102,115]. In a recent study, *Jensen* et al. [56] have monitored the effects of chemotherapy by use of localized proton spectroscopy (STEAM technique). The major finding is a clearly abnormal

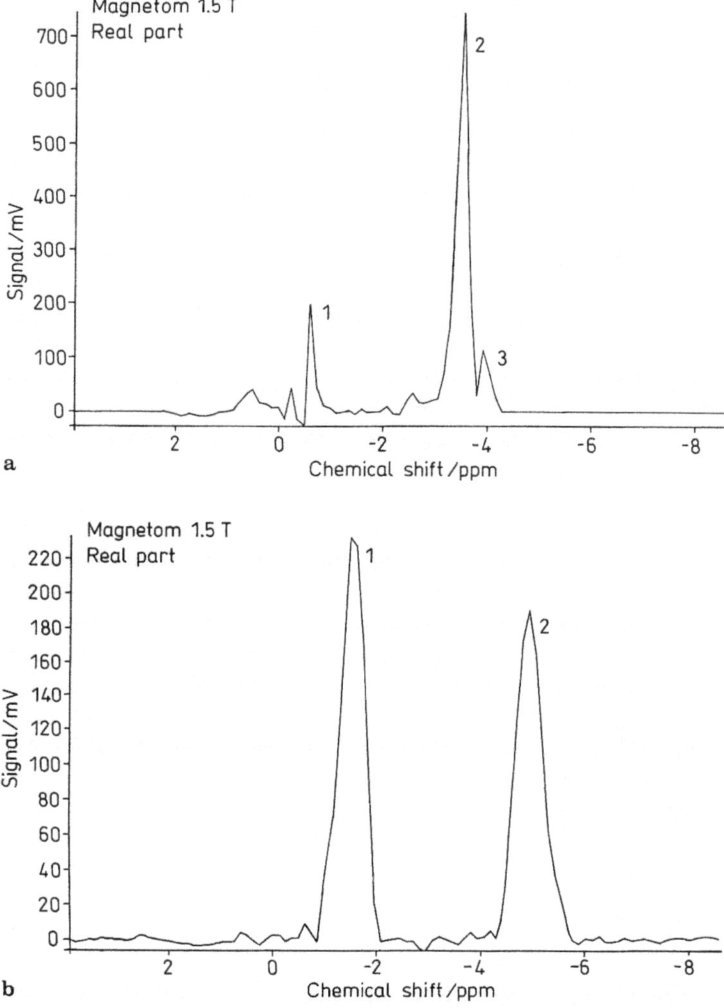

Fig. 8 a, b. Spectra obtained with the STEAM technique **a** from a cubic VOI in tibial (fatty) bone marrow (①), "water" resonance) in a normal volunteer, **b** from iliac bone marrow in the same volunteer, give for comparison. The "relative water content" is markedly increased compared to normal tibial marrow. In tibial bone marrow three resonances could be resolved: "water" protons (①), —CH_2— groups of lipid (②), and —CH_3— groups of lipid (③). (From [57]).

spectral pattern in all 13 patients with leukemia at the time of diagnosis with a subsequent reappearance of the fat resonance during successful chemotherapy (as seen in Fig. 9). Indeed the sensitivity of the STEAM technique seems to be high since alterations in the content of bone marrow fat can be detected shortly after the start of erythropoietin treatment in patients with anemia caused by end-stage renal disease [57]. Thus, CSI methods and localized proton spectroscopy may

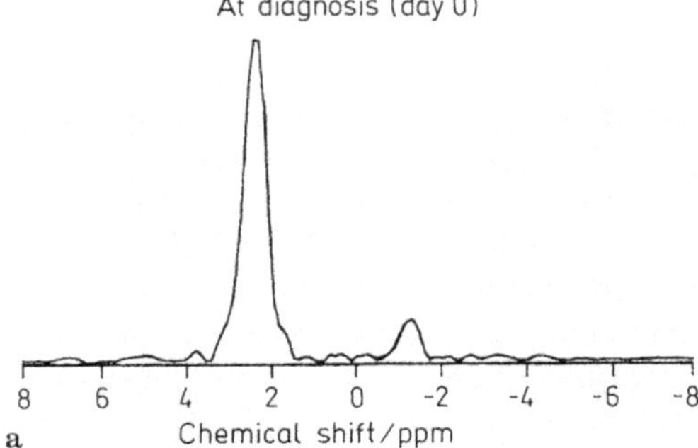

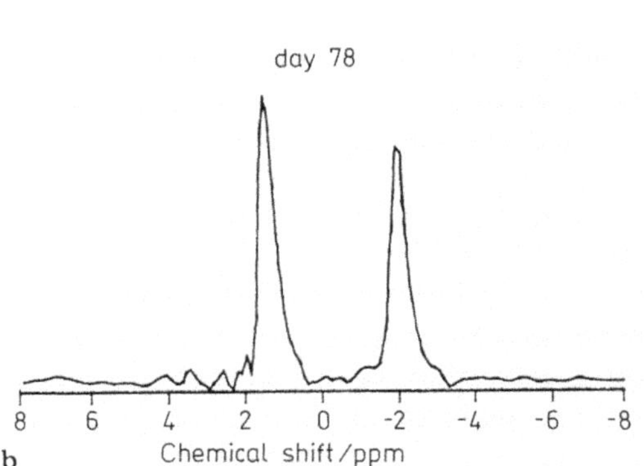

Fig. 9 a, b. Two proton spectra acquired with the STEAM technique from a cubic VOI in the left iliac bone marrow of a patient with acute myeloid leukemia (AML) in relation to treatment with chemotherapy **a** at the time of diagnosis (day 0) and **b** 78 days after start of chemotherapy (bone marrow in complete remission). The water and fat resonances could be identified (the water resonance was assigned as follows: 2.4 ppm at day 0, and 1.5 ppm at day 78). The T1 relaxation times of the water resonance in the iliac bone marrow spectra were: day 0, 1050 ms and day 78, 250 ms. Note the increase in peak area of the fat resonance and the decrease in T1 value of the water resonance in relation to induction of remission. (From [56])

supplement histological bone marrow examinations in regions inaccessible to biopsy.

Also, focal infiltrative bone marrow disease could well be evaluated with CSI methods and a number of conditions could benefit with respect to clinical management: lymphoma, skeletal metastases, and primary skeletal cancer [91]. The beneficial effects could be both diagnostic and improved possibilities for monitoring of treatment during follow-up examinations [56].

The use of CSI methods in benign bone marrow disorders seems to hold a great potential, and a substantial amount of data from investigations of avascular bone necrosis has been reported [72, 76]. The results from CSI investigations may aid the comparison of different treatment methods in the future [76].

9 Oncology

One of the clinically most interesting potential applications of spectroscopy is the noninvasive monitoring of treatment effects during cancer therapy. During the last decade an extensive data base of knowledge has been provided from a large number of in vitro cell suspensions or in vivo animal models [35, 39, 37]. Clinical studies of humans have been concentrated on superficially located tumors investigated with phosphorus spectroscopy (using surface coil techniques). In 12 out of 14 patients *Ross* [94] observed clearly abnormal phosphorus spectral patterns in osteosarcomas and lymphomas, as compared with skeletal muscle. The spectral changes primarily consisted of changes in the PME and PDE resonances. A metabolic response to therapy was detected in two patients [94]. *Semmler* et al. [101] have studied the effects of chemotherapy as well as radiation therapy on large superficial tumors in 23 patients using a simple surface coil technique for volume selection. This study included both long-term and short-term follow-up examinations during treatment. The results indicate that early changes in the high-energy phosphorus metabolism can be detected after the start of treatment. One finding has been an increase in the sum of PCr and Pi, another finding was an increase in the PCr to Pi ratio. There seem, however, to be large variations in treatment response between patients as well as between tumors of identical histological type. So the clinical value of these investigations is not clear at present. On the other hand, the possibilities for serial monitoring of treatment response in vivo opens up a new research area where new methods for volume selections combined with multinuclear (both phosphorus and proton) spectroscopy may add important clinical information. Techniques with capacity for high-quality selection of small tissue volumes ($< 1\,\text{cm}^3$) and methods for absolute quantification of metabolite concentrations are needed especially when the tumor volumes decrease during treatment. Localized water suppressed proton spectroscopy of superficial tumors (i.e., extremity tumors) have not been reported so far, but may be a new area for clinical spectroscopic investigations. An interesting approach is spectroscopic studies of distribution and metabolism of fluorine (^{19}F)-labeled drugs [116]. *Semmler* et al. [100] have studied the metabolism of 5-fluorouracil in liver tumors in eight patients using a surface coil technique. This study proves that more detailed data of the metabolism during chemotherapy can be obtained with the use of ^{19}F-labeled compounds in spite of the crude localization technique employed.

10 General Discussion and Future Trends

The main question of whether MR spectroscopy is likely to become relevant in terms of routine clinical application and diagnostic investigation remains open. The use of MR spectroscopy in a clinical environment has progressed at a slow rate compared to the application of high-resolution MRI. The main reasons for this may be the higher technical demands of the spectroscopic methods combined with the more complex interpretation of the spectroscopic results [1]. Increased technical developments during the last 5 years together with a major increase in the number of high-field MR scanners have provided a firm base for a rapid expansion in clinical research. The very recent development of experimental whole body spectrometers operating at 4 T [15, 45] together with new double spin echo methods for volume selection may further advance the application to new organ systems and pathological conditions [20, 82]. It is now possible to obtain reliable and precise results from humans in vivo at clinically installed MR imagers [48], and areas which hold promise for future clinical use of spectroscopy have been identified for phosphorus spectroscopy (skeletal muscle) as well as for proton spectroscopy (brain, liver, and bone marrow). Technical problems regarding standard tests of volume selection and methods for actual metabolite quantification will probably be further clarified in the near future. Initiatives for international cooperation in providing appropriate test phantoms for quality assessment of clinical spectroscopic methods have been taken with the EEC Concerted Action on tissue characterization by MRI and MRS [84]. Results from quality control studies of spectroscopic methods on the EEC phantoms have been reported [109, 60]. The biological problems include the inherent low sensitivity of MR spectroscopy which causes limited possibilities for reasonable spatial resolution ($< 1\,\mathrm{cm}^3$) compared to MRI ($< 1\,\mathrm{mm}^3$) within a clinically acceptable measurement time. Thus, the forthcoming research in clinical spectroscopy must investigate medical questions which can be answered within reasonable technical demands. At the present stage further studies in normal subjects especially with emphasis on characterizing the variation in spectroscopic data with age, sex, and different location within given tissues are needed. Furthermore, research clarifying the connection between human research and spectroscopic results obtained from animal models are warranted. Another aspect of the coming research in clinical research will be the educational process for the staff that conduct the spectroscopic examinations. Whereas MRI provides results similar to computerized tomography (CT), MRS provides rather complex chemical information, and educational programs for physicians are important in order to secure a high-quality standard in future clinical routine [1].

In conclusion, we believe that in vivo MR spectroscopy of human beings at the present state remains a very powerful research modality. Some of the clinical applications of MR spectroscopy are very close to clinical routine (skeletal muscle disease). As a preliminary answer to the question of clinical relevance for a major percentage of the patient population we see some definite trends towards clinical routine in the future. As mentioned throughout the present review a substantial amount of clinical as well as basic research is needed before any definite conclusions about the value of MR spectroscopy on patient diagnosis and treatment can be drawn.

References

1. Aisen AM, Chenevert TL (1989) MR spectroscopy: clinical perspective. Radiology 173:593–599
2. Angus PW, Dixon RM, Rajagopalan B, Ryley NG, Simpson KJ, Peters TJ, Jewell DP, Radda GK (1990) A study of patients with alcoholic liver disease by 31 P nuclear magnetic resonance spectroscopy. Clin Sci 78:33–38
3. Argov Z, Bank WJ, Maris J, Chance B (1987) Muscle energy metabolism in McArdle's syndrome by in vivo phosphorus magnetic resonance spectroscopy. Neurology 37:1720–1724
4. Argov Z, Bank WJ, Maris, J, Eleff S, Kennaway NG, Olson RE, Chance B (1986) Treatment of mitochondrial myopathy due to complex III dificiency with vitamins K3 and C:A 31 P-NMR follow-up study. Ann Neurol 19:598–602
5. Argov Z, Bank WJ, Maris J, Leigh JS Jr, Chance B (1987) Muscle energy metabolism in human phosphofructokinase deficiency as recorded by 31 P nuclear magnetic resonance spectroscopy. Ann Neurol 22:46–51
6. Argov Z, Bank WJ, Maris J, Peterson P, Chance B (1987) Bioenergetic heterogeneity of human mitochondrial myopathies: phosphorus magnetic resonance spectroscopy study. Neurology 37:257–262
7. Arnold DL, Matthews PM, Francis G, Antel J (1990) Proton magnetic resonance spectroscopy of human brain in vivo in the evaluation of multiple sclerosis: assessment of the load of disease. Magn Reson Med 14:154–159
8. Arnold DL, Bore PJ, Radda GK, Styles P, Taylor DJ (1984) Excessive intracellular acidosis of skeletal muscle on exercise in a patient with a post-viral exhaustion/fatigue syndrome. A 31 P nuclear magnetic resonance study. Lancet 1:1367–1369
9. Aue WP (1986) Localization methods for in vivo nuclear magnetic resonance spectroscopy. Reviews of Magn Reson Med 1:21–72
10. Baker AJ, Carson PJ, Miller RG, Weiner MW (1989) Investigations of muscle bioenergetics with 31 P NMR. Invest Radiol 24:1001–1005
11. Barany M, Langer BG, Glick RP, Venkatasubramanian PN, Wilbur AC, Spigos DG (1988) In vivo H-1 spectroscopy in humans at 1.5 T. Radiology 167:839–844
12. Barany M, Siegel IM, Venkatasubramanian PN, Mok E, Wilbur AC (1989) Human leg neuromuscular diseases: P-31 MR spectroscopy. Radiology 172:503–508
13. Barany M, Spigos DG, Mok E, Venkatasubramanian PN, Wilbur AC, Langer BG (1987) High resolution proton magnetic resonance spectroscopy of human brain and liver. Magn Reson Imaging 5:393–398
14. Barany M, Venkatasubramanian PN, Mok E, Siegel IM, Abraham E, Wycliffe ND, Mafee MF (1989) Quantitative and qualitative fat analysis in human leg muscle of neuromuscular diseases by 1 H MR spectroscopy in vivo. Magn Reson Med 10:210–226
15. Barfuss H, Fischer H, Hentschel D, Ladebeck R, Vetter J (1988) Whole-body MR imaging and spectroscopy with a 4-T system. Radiology 169:811–816
16. Berkelbach van der Sprenkel JW, Luyten PR, van Rijen PC, Tulleken CA, Den Hollander JA (1988) Cerebral lactate detected by regional proton magnetic resonance spectroscopy in a patient with cerebral infarction. Stroke 19:1556–1560
17. Blackledge MJ, Rajagopalan B, Oberhaensli RD, Bolas NM, Styles P, Radda GK (1987) Quantitative studies of human cardiac metabolism by 31 P rotating-frame NMR. Proc Natl Acad Sci USA. 84:4283–4287
18. Bore-PJ (1985) The role of magnetic resonance spectroscopy in clinical medicine. Magn Reson Imaging 3:407–413
19. Boska MD, Moussavi RS, Carson PJ, Weiner MW, Miller RG (1990) The metabolic basis of recovery after fatiguing exercise of human muscle. Neurology 40:240–244
20. Boska MD, Hubesch B, Meyerhoff DJ, Twieg DB, Karczmar GS, Matson GB, Weiner MW (1990) Comparison of 31 P MRS and 1 H MRI at 1.5 and 2.0 T. Magn Reson Med 13:228–238
21. Bottomley PA (1989) Human in vivo NMR spectroscopy in diagnostic medicine: clinical tool or research probe? Radiology 170:1–15
22. Bottomley PA (1985) Noninvasive study of high-energy phosphate metabolism in human heart by depth-resolved 31 P NMR spectroscopy. Science 229:769–772
23. Bottomley PA, Charles HC, Roemer PB, Flamig D, Engeseth H, Edelstein WA, Mueller OM (1988) Human in vivo phosphate metabolite imaging with 31 P NMR. Magn Reson Med 7:319–336
24. Bottomley PA, Drayer BP, Smith LS (1986) Chronic adult cerebral infarction studied by phosphorus NMR spectroscopy. Radiology 160:763–766

25. Bottomley PA, Forster TB, Darrow RD (1984) Depth-resolved surface-coil spectroscopy (DRESS) for in vivo H-1, P-31 and C-13 NMR. J Magn Reson 59:338–342
26. Bottomley PA, Hart HR Jr, Edelstein WA, Schenck JF, Smith LS, Leue WM, Mueller OM, Redington RW (1984) Anatomy and metabolism of the normal human brain studied by magnetic resonance at 1.5 Tesla. Radiology 150:441–446
27. Bottomley PA, Herfkens RJ, Smith LS, Bashore TM (1987) Altered phosphate metabolism in myocardial infarction: P-31 MR spectroscopy. Radiology 165:703–707
28. Bottomley PA, Smith LS, Brazzamano S, Hedlund LW, Redington RW, Herfkens RJ, (1987) The fate of inorganic phosphate and pH in regional myocardial ischemia and infarction: a noninvasive 31 P NMR study. Magn Reson Med 5:129–142
29. Brateman L (1986) Chemical shift imaging: a review. AJR 146:971–980
30. Brink HF, Buschmann MD, Rosen BR (1989) NMR chemical shift imaging. Comput Med Imaging Graph 13:93–104
31. Bruhn H, Frahm J, Gyngell ML, Merboldt KD, Hanicke W, Sauter R, Hamburger C (1989) Noninvasive differentiation of tumors with use of localized H-1 MR spectroscopy in vivo: initial experience in patients with cerebral tumors. Radiology 172:541–548
32. Bruhn H, Frahm J, Gyngell ML, Merboldt KD, Hanicke W, Sauter R (1989) Cerebral metabolism in man after acute stroke: new observations using localized proton NMR spectroscopy. Magn Reson Med 9:126–131
33. Cady EB, Costello AM, Dawson MJ, Delphy DT, Hope PL, Reynolds EO, Tofts PS, Wilkie DR (1983) Non-invasive investigation of cerebral metabolism in newborn infants by phosphorus nuclear magnetic resonance spectroscopy. Lancet i:1059–1062
34. Chance B, Younkin DP, Kelley R, Bank WJ, Berkowitz HD, Argov Z, Donlon E, Boden B, McCully K, Buist NM (1986) Magnetic resonance spectroscopy of normal and diseased muscles. Am J Med Genet 25:659–679
35. Cohen JS (1988) Phospholipid and energy metabolism of cancer cells monitored by 31 P magnetic resonance spectroscopy: possible clinical significance. Mayo Clin Proc 63:1199–1207
36. Cox IJ, Kay JDS, Anderson SBT, Bryant DJ, Ross BD (1987) Liver versus kidney for acid-base control? The Pitts–Atkinson controversy re-examined by hepatic 31 P MR spectroscopy in man. Sixth Annual Meeting of the Society of Magnetic Resonance in Medicine, New York, Abstract book, p 984
37. Daly PF, Cohen JS (1989) Magnetic resonance spectroscopy of tumors and potential in vivo clinical applications: a review. Cancer Res 49:770–779
38. Dixon WT (1984) Simple proton spectroscopic imaging. Radiology 153:189–194
39. Evanochko WT, Ng TC, Glickson JD (1984) Application of in vivo NMR spectroscopy to cancer. Magn Reson Med 1:508–534
40. Frahm J, Bruhn H, Gyngell ML, Merboldt KD, Hanicke W, Sauter R (1989) Localized high-resolution proton NMR spectroscopy using stimulated echoes: initial applications to human brain in vivo. Magn Reson Med 9:79–93
41. Frahm J, Bruhn H, Gyngell ML, Merboldt KD, Hanicke W, Sauter R (1989b) Localized proton NMR spectroscopy in different regions of the human brain in vivo. Relaxation times and concentrations of cerebral metabolites. Magn Reson Med 11:47–63
42. Frahm J, Haase A, Hanicke W, Matthaei D, Bomsdorf H, Helzel T (1985) Chemical shift selective MR imaging using a whole-body magnet. Radiology 156:441–444
43. Gordon PJ, Hanley PE, Shaw D, Gadian DG, Radda GK, Styles P, Bore PJ, Chan L (1980) Localization of metabolites in animals using P-31 topical magnetic resonance. Nature 287:367–368
44. Hands LJ, Bore PJ, Galloway G, Morris PJ, Radda GK (1986) Muscle metabolism in patients with peripheral vascular disease investigated by 31 P nuclear magnetic resonance spectroscopy. Clin Sci 71:283–290
45. Hardy CJ, Bottomley PA, Roemer PB, Redington RW (1988) Rapid 31 P spectroscopy on a 4-T whole-body system. Magn Reson Med 8:104–109
46. Hayes DJ, Taylor DJ, Bore PJ, Hilton-Jones D, Arnold DL, Squier MV, Gent AE, Radda GK (1987) An unusual metabolic myopathy: a malate-aspartate shuttle defect. J Neurol Sci 82:27–39
47. Heiken JP, Lee JKT, Dixon WT (1985) Fatty infiltration of the liver: evaluation by proton spectroscopic imaging. Radiology 157:707–710
48. Henriksen O, Larsson H, Jensen KM (1990) In vivo H-1 spectroscopy of human brain at 1.5 Tesla. Preliminary experience at a clinical installation. Acta Radiol 31:181–186
49. Henriksen O, Wieslander S, Gjerris F, Jensen KM (1991) In vivo H-1 spectroscopy of human intracranial tumours at 1.5 Tesla. Preliminary experience at clinical installation. Acta Radiol 32:95–99

50. Hope PL, Costello AM, Cady EB, Delphy DT, Tofts PS, Chu A, Hamilton PA, Reynolds EO, Wilkie DR (1984) Cerebral energy metabolism studied with phosphorus NMR spectroscopy in normal and birth-asphyxiated infants. Lancet ii:366–370
51. Hope PL, Reynolds EO (1985) Investigation of cerebral energy metabolism in newborn infants by phosphorus nuclear magnetic resonance spectroscopy. Clin Perinatol 12:261–275
52. Hubesch B, Marinier DS, Hetherington HP, Twieg DB, Weiner MW (1989) Clinical MRS studies of the brain. Invest Radiol 24:1039–1042
53. Hubesch B, Marinier DS, Roth K, Meyerhoff DJ, Matson GB, Weiner MW (1990) P-31 MR spectroscopy of normal human brain and brain tumors. Radiology 174:401–409
54. Irving MG, Brooks WM, Brereton IM, Galloway GJ, Field J, Bell JR, Harris MG, Baddeley H, Doddrell DM (1987) Use of high resolution in vivo volume selected 1 H-magnetic resonance spectroscopy to investigate leukemia in humans. Cancer Res 47:3901–3906
55. Jensen KE, Jakobsen J, Thomsen C, Henriksen O (1990a) Improved energy kinetics following high protein diet in McArdle's syndrom. Acta Neurol Scand 81:499–503
56. Jensen KE, Jensen M, Sørensen PG, Thomsen C, Karle H, Henriksen O (1990b) Localized in vivo proton spectroscopy of the bone marrow in patients with leukaemia. Magn Reson Imaging 8(6):779–789
57. Jensen KE, Stenver D, Jensen M, Grundtvig P, Thomsen C, Karle H, Henriksen O, Nielsen B (1990) Effects of recombinant human erythropoietin on the bone marrow monitored by magnetic resonance spectroscopy in patients with end-stage renal disease. Magn Reson Imaging 8:237–243
58. Jensen KE, Jacobsen S, Thomsen C, Andersen RB, Henriksen O (1988) In vivo 31 P-magnetic resonance spectroscopy during exercise in patients with primary fibromyalgia (abstract). Radiology 169(P):238
59. Jensen KE, Thomsen C, Henriksen O (1988) In vivo measurement of intracellular pH in human brain during different tensions of carbon dioxide in arterial blood. A 31 P-NMR study. Acta Physiol Scand 134:295–298
60. Jensen KM, Thomsen C, Podo F, Henriksen O (1988) First experience with a new test object for quality control of volume selective spectroscopy. Seventh Annual Meeting of the Society of Magnetic Resonance in Medicine, San Francisco, p 59
61. Keller U, Oberhaensli R, Huber P, Widmer LK, Aue WP, Hassink RI, Muller S, Seelig J (1985) Phosphocreatine content and intracellular pH of calf muscle measured by phosphorus NMR spectroscopy in occlusive arterial disease of the legs. Eur J Clin Invest 15:382–388
62. Lane RJ, Arnold DL, Bore PJ, Taylor DJ, Radda GK, Walton J (1987) 31 P-NMR studies in patients with exertional muscle pain syndrome (EMPS) responding to verapamil (letter). Muscle Nerve 10:183–184
63. Larsson HBW, Christiansen P, Jensen M, Frederiksen J, Heltberg A, Olese J, Henriksen O (to be published) Localized in vivo proton spectroscopy in the brain of patients with multiple sclerosis. Magn Reson Med
64. Lee JK, Dixon WT, Ling D, Levitt RG, Murphy WA Jr (1984) Fatty infiltration of the liver: demonstration by proton spectroscopic imaging. Preliminary observations. Radiology 153:195–201
65. Lee JK, Heiken JP, Dixon WT (1985) Detection of hepatic metastases by proton spectroscopic imaging. Work in progress. Radiology 156:429–433
66. Lenkinski RE (1989) Clinical magnetic resonance spectroscopy: a critical evaluation. Invest Radiol 24:1034–1038
67. Levine SR, Welch KMA, Helpern JA, Bruce R, Smith MB (1987) Clinical investigation of ischemic stroke by serial 31-phosphorus NMR spectroscopy (abstract). Sixth Annual Meeting of the Society of Magnetic Resonance in Medicine, New York, Book of abstracts, p 536
68. Luyten PR, den Hollander JA, van der Knaap S, Valk J (1988) P-31 and H-1 MR spectroscopic examination of patients with white-mater disorders (abstract). Radiology 169(P):41
69. Luyten PR, Anderson CM, den Hollander JA (1987) 1 H NMR relaxation measurements of human tissues in situ by spatially resolved spectroscopy. Magn Reson Med 4:431–440
70. Luyten PR, den Hollander JA (1986) 1 H MR spatially resolved spectroscopy of human tissues in situ. Magn Reson Imaging 4:237–239
71. Mancini DM, Ferraro N, Tuchler M, Chance B, Wilson JR (1988) Detection of abnormal calf muscle metabolism in patients with heart failure using phosphorus-31 nuclear magnetic resonance. Am J Cardiol 62:1234–1240
72. Matthaei D, Frahm J, Haase A, Schuster R, Bomsdorf H (1985) Chemical-shift-selective magnetic-resonance imaging of avascular necrosis of the femoral head. Lancet i:370–371
73. Meyerhoff DJ, Boska MD, Thomas AM, Weiner MW (1989) Alcoholic liver disease: quantitative image-guided P-31 MR spectroscopy. Radiology 173:393–400

74. Miller RG, Boska MD, Moussavi RS, Carson PJ, Weiner MW (1988) 31P nuclear magnetic resonance studies of high energy phosphates and pH in human muscle fatigue. Comparison of aerobic and anaerobic exercise. J Clin Invest 81:1190–1196
75. Miller RG, Giannini D, Milner-Brown HS, Layzer RB, Koretsky AP, Hooper D, Weiner MW (1987) Effects of fatiguing exercise on high-energy phosphates, force, and EMG: evidence for three phases of recovery. Muscle Nerve 10:810–821
76. Mitchell DG, Joseph PM, Fallon M, Hickey W, Kressel HY, Rao VM, Steinberg ME, Dalinka MK (1987) Chemical-shift MR imaging of the femoral head: an in vitro study of normal hips and hips with avascular necrosis. AJR 148:1159–1164
77. Narayana PA, Jackson EF, Hazle JD, Fotedar LK, Kulkarni MV, Flamig DP (1989) In vivo localized proton spectroscopic studies of human gastrocnemius muscle. Magn Reson Med 12:259–260
78. Narayana PA, Slopis JM, Jackson EF, Hazle JD, Kulkarni MV, Butler IJ (1989) In vivo muscle magnetic resonance spectroscopy in a family with mitochondrial cytopathy: a defect in fat metabolism. Magn Reson Imaging 7:133–139
79. Nunnally RL, Babcock EE, Vaughan JT, Klein DL, Bonte FJ, Walker-Batson D. (1987) Examination of brain metabolism in chronic stroke patients: a phosphorus-31 nuclear magnetic resonance study (abstract). Sixth Annual Meeting of the Society of Magnetic Resonance in Medicine, New York, Book of abstracts, p 538
80. Oberhaensli RD, Galloway GJ, Taylor DJ, Bore PJ, Radda GK (1986) Assessment of human liver metabolism by phosphorus-31 magnetic resonance spectroscopy. Br J Radiol 59:695–699
81. Ordidge RJ, Connelly A, Lohman JAB (1986) Image-selected in vivo spectroscopy (ISIS). A new Technique for spatially selective NMR spectroscopy. J Magn Reson 66:283–294
82. Ortendahl DA (1988) Whole-body MR imaging and spectroscopy at 4 T: where do we go from here? (editorial). Radiology 169:864–865
83. Osbakken M, Ligeti L, Huddell J, Duska C, Ponomarenko I, Chance B (1989) In vivo myocardial bioenergetics during acute volume and/or pressure loading in a canine model: a 31P NMR study. Cardiology 76:405–417
84. Podo F (1988) Tissue characterization by MRI: a multidisciplinary and multi-centre challenge today (editorial). Magn Reson Imaging 6:173–174
85. Quistorff B, Nielsen S, Thomsen C, Jensen KE, Henriksen O (1990) A simple calf muscle ergometer for use in a standard whole-body MR-scanner. Magn Reson Med 13:444–449
86. Radda GK (1986) The use of NMR spectroscopy for the understanding of disease. Science 233:640–645
87. Radda GK, Taylor DJ, Arnold DL (1985) Investigation of human mitochondrial myopathies by phosphorus magnetic resonance spectroscopy. Biochem Soc Trans 13:654
88. Rajagopalan B, Blackedge MJ, McKenna WJ, Bolas N, Radda GK (1987) Measurement of phosphocreatine to ATP ratio in normal and diseased human heart by 31P magnetic resonance spectroscopy using the rotating frame-depth selection technique. Ann NY Acad Sci 508:321–332.
89. Rajagopalan B, Bristow JD, Radda GK (1989) Measurement of transmural distribution of phosphorus metabolites in the pig heart by 31P magnetic resonance spectroscopy. Cardiovasc Res 23:1015–1026
90. Rajagopalan B, Conway MA, Massie B, Radda GK (1988) Alterations of skeletal muscle metabolism in humans studied by phosphorus 31 magnetic resonance spectroscopy in congestive heart failure. Am J Cardiol 62:53E–57E
91. Redmond OM, Stack JP, Dervan PA, Hurson BJ, Carney DN, Ennis JT (1989) Osteosarcoma: use of MR imaging and MR spectroscopy in clinical decision making. Radiology 172:811–815
92. Richards TL, Davis CA, Barker BR, Beinert WD, Genant HK (1987) Lipid/water ratio of bone marrow measured by phase-encoded proton nuclear magnetic resonance spectroscopy. Invest Radiol 22:741–746
93. Rosen BR, Fleming DM, Kushner DC, Zaner KS, Buxton RB, Bennet WP, Wismer GL, Brady TJ (1988) Hematologic bone marrow disorders: quantitative chemical shift MR imaging. Radiology 169:799–804
94. Ross BD (1988) The current state of clinical magnetic resonance spectroscopy with phosphorus-31: a view from Hammersmith. Magn Reson Med Biol 1:81–98
95. Schaefer S, Camacho SA, Gober J, Obregon RG, DeGroot MA, Botvinick EH, Massie B, Weiner MW (1989) Response of myocardial metabolites to graded regional ischemia: 31P NMR spectroscopy of porcine myocardium in vivo. Circ Res 64:968–976
96. Schertz LD, Lee JKT, Heiken JP, Molina PL, Totty WG (1989) Proton spectroscopic imaging (Dixon method) of the liver: clinical utility. Radiology 173:401–405

97. Segebarth CM, Baleriaux DF, Arnold DL, Luyten PR, den Hollander JA (1987) MR image-guided P-31 MR spectroscopy in the evaluation of brain tumor treatment. Radiology 165:215–219
98. Segebarth CM, Baleriaux DF, de Beer R, van Ormondt-D, Marien A, Luyten PR, den Hollander JA (1989) 1H image-guided localized 31P MR spectroscopy of human brain: quantitative analysis of 31P MR spectra measured on volunteers and on intracranial tumor patients. Magn Reson Med 11:349–366
99. Segebarth CM, Baleriaux DF, Luyten PR, den Hollander JA (1990) Detection of metabolic heterogeneity of human intracranial tumors in vivo by 1H NMR spectroscopic imaging. Magn Reson Med 13:62–76
100. Semmler W, Bachert-Baumann P, Guckel F, Ermark F, Schlag P, Lorenz WJ, van Kaick G (1990) Real-time follow-up of 5-fluorouracil metabolism in the liver of tumor patients by means of F-19 MR spectroscopy. Radiology 174:141–145
101. Semmler W, Gademann G, Bachert-Baumann P, Zabel HJ, Lorenz WJ, van Kaick G (1988) Monitoring human tumor response to therapy by means of P-31 MR spectroscopy. Radiology 166:533–539
102. Sepponen RE, Sipponen JT, Tanttu JI (1984) A method for chemical shift imaging: demonstration of bone marrow involvement with proton chemical shift imaging. J Comput Assist Tomogr 8:585–587
103. Styles P, Scott CA, Radda GK (1985) A method for localizing high-resolution NMR spectra from human subjects. Magn Reson Med 2:402–409
104. Taylor DJ, Brosnan MJ, Arnold DL, Bore PJ, Styles P, Walton J, Radda GK (1988) Ca2 + -ATPase deficiency in a patient with an exertional muscle pain syndrome. J Neurol Neurosurg Psychiatry 51:1425–1433
105. Taylor DJ, Styles P, Matthews PM, Arnold DA, Gadian DG, Bore P, Radda GK (1986) Energetics of human muscle: exercise-induced ATP depletion. Magn Reson Med 3:44–54
106. Terrier F, Vock P, Cotting J, Ladebeck R, Reichen J, Hentschel D (1989) Effect of intravenous fructose on the P-31 MR spectrum of the liver: dose response in healthy volunteers. Radiology 171:557–563
107. Thomsen C, Jensen KE, Achten E, Henriksen O (1988) In vivo MR Imaging and ^{31}P-spectroscopy of large human brain tumours at 1.5 Tesla. Acta Radiol 29:77–82
108. Thomsen C, Jensen KE, Henriksen O (1989) 31P NMR measurements of T2 relaxation times of metabolites in human skeletal muscle in vivo. Magn Reson Imaging 7:557–559
109. Thomsen C, Jensen KE, Jensen M, Olsen ER, Henriksen O (1990) MR pulse sequences for selective relaxation time measurements. A phantom study. Magn Reson Imaging 8:43–50
110. Twieg DB, Meyerhoff DJ, Hubesch B, Roth K, Marinier DS, Boska MD, Gober JR, Schaefer S, Weiner MW (1989) Phosphorus-31 magnetic resonance spectroscopy in humans by spectroscopic imaging: localized spectroscopy and metabolite imaging. Magn Reson Med 12:291–305
111. van Rijen PC, Luyten PR, van der Sprenkel JW, Kraaier V, van Huffelen AC, Tulleken CA, den Hollander JA (1989) 1H and 31P NMR measurement of cerebral lactate, high-energy phosphate levels, and pH in humans during voluntary hyperventilation: associated EEG, capnographic, and Doppler findings. Magn Reson Med 10:182–193
112. Weiner MW (1988) The promise of magnetic resonance spectroscopy for medical diagnosis. Invest Radiol 23:253–261
113. Wiener DH, Fink LI, Maris J, Jones RA, Chance B, Wilson JR (1986) Abnormal skeletal muscle bioenergetics during exercise in patients with heart failure: role of reduced muscle blood flow. Circulation 73:1127–1136
114. Williams DM, Fencil L,. Chenevert TL (1990) Peripheral arterial occlusive disease: P-31 MR spectroscopy of calf muscle. Radiology 175:381–385
115. Wismer GL, Rosen BR, Buxton R, Stark DD, Brady TJ (1985) Chemical shift imaging of bone marrow: preliminary experience. AJR 145:1031–1037
116. Wolf W, Silver MS, Albright MJ, Weber H, Reichardt U, Sauter R (1987) A non-invasive study of drug metabolism in patients as studied by 19-F NMR spectroscopy of 5-fluorouracil. Ann N Y Acad Sci 508:491–493
117. Young IR (1990) Magnetic resonance: boundless possibilities ⋯ or possible boundaries. Br J Radiol 63:1–13

Image Contour Spread in Computed Tomography

S. Tabakoff

1 Introduction

Problems of image contour spread in roentgenology are well known. They concern the influence of different apparatus, X-ray, photo, and optical parameters on the image unsharpness and on the corresponding spatial resolution [3, 14]. In conventional roentgenology, there exist different methods for decrease in image unsharpness that is, decrease in their contour spread. This fact, combined with the specific features of the X-ray image, causes spread width (the transition layer width between the images of two contiguous structures) to be normally below 1 mm, this having no substantial effect on diagnostical interpretation.

In computed tomography (CT) images are indirectly formed after mathematical reconstruction of X-ray projections, obtained at irradiation of the object from different angles. Each X-ray projection is a summary absorption of X-rays by all objects lying between the X-ray table and the detector system. That is why in the reconstruction process there is a great mutual influence among calculated absorption values (density units, HU) of different structures building the object. Thus the density of each pixel from the CT image contains data not only about the corresponding microvolume (voxel) of the object, but also data about neighboring microvolumes. This results in obtaining additional "calculative" poor clarity, which exceeds considerably the poor clarity in conventional roentgenology

Using various image processing techniques decreases to a certain degree the calculative unsharpness, but this process is strongly influenced by the type of processing as well as by some apparatus parameters. As these particularities of

Department of Roentgenology, Higher Medical Institute—Plovdiv, boul. V. Aprilov 15, 4000 Plovdiv, Bulgaria

Frontiers in European Radiology, Vol. 8
Eds. Baert/Heuck
© Springer-Verlag, Berlin Heidelberg 1991

CT image often cause diagnostical problems, especially in diagnosing small objects, we examined the practical contour spread width of images in CT and its dependence on different apparatus parameters.

2 Materials and Methods

Examinations are carried out on rotational CT apparatuses from the third generation. Basically CT scanner type CE10000 (1024 + 11 xenon detectors) from the firm CGR is used, having the following parameters:

— Matrix of 256 × 256 or 512 × 512 and reconstruction fields of 130 mm, 260 mm, 290 mm, and 520 mm ensuring pixel sizes from 0.25 to 2 mm
— Scanning times of 3.4 s, 6.8 s, and 13.6 s, ensuring, correspondingly, 512, 1024, and 2048 projections
— Reconstructive filters: low frequency (density), high frequency (spatial), and intermediate (standard)
— Slice widths of 10 mm, 5 mm, and 1.5 mm
— X-ray radiation with 120 kVp and tube current from 40 to 100 mA with respect to the dynamic range of detectors at the corresponding slice width.

AAPM phantom type 74–410 and our phantom are used as test objects. The spread of the sharp density edge, formed by two contiguous homogeneous bodies, or by a body and its surrounding homogeneous medium, is examined. As spread width is measured the linearly varying part of the densoprofile between the two constant densities of the bodies forms the density transition (Fig. 1a, b). Two types of transition are examined with a density gradient between 30 and 120 HU and between 800 and 1200 HU. The width of the transition layer was defined at all apparatus parameters, in two places at the scanning surface (near to the

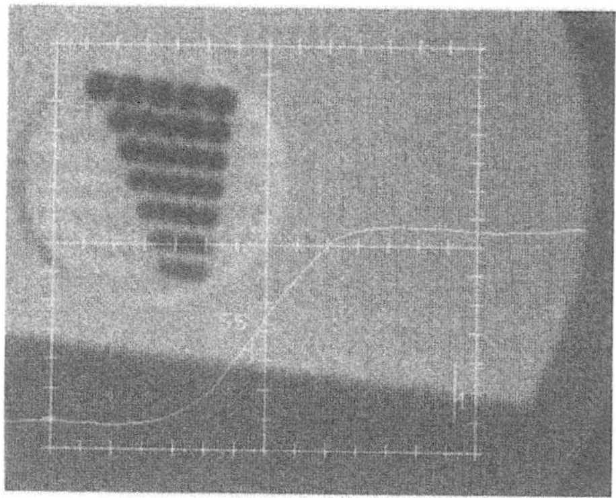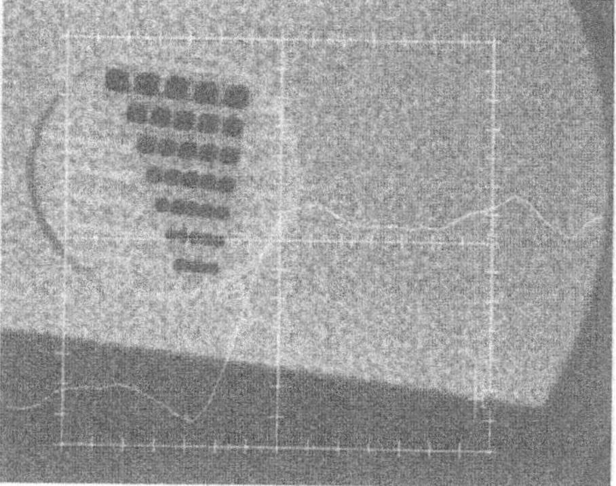

a   b

Fig. 1 a, b. Densoprofile determination of the image spread for a sharp density transition. **a** Increased spread (widened transition layer)—256 × 256 matrix, low-frequency reconstruction filter. **b** Decreased spread (narrowed transition layer)—512 × 512 matrix, high-frequency reconstruction filter

center and near to the periphery), and at three measuring positions—horizontally, vertically, and along the diagonal of the matrix. The whole study was performed over 2 years with two different X-ray tubes—at the beginning and at the end of their exploitation period. The basic results are verified also on CT apparatuses produced by Siemens and Philips. The values obtained are averaged.

3 Results

The examination and analysis of over 5000 transition layers showed that spread width is mainly influenced by pixel size, type of reconstruction filter, slice width, and density gradient. In accordance with them, spread width varies from 0.7 to 7 mm. The values averaged at scanning time 6.8 s for slice thickness 10 mm and 5 mm are shown on Fig. 2a, b. Results at 1.5 mm slice thickness are almost the same as these at 5-mm slice thickness (or CE10000).

Based on the above values, the averaged results vary as follows:

— Increase in scanning time (13.6 s) leads to decrease in spread width of 0.5–0.7 mm.
— Decrease in scanning time (3.4 s) leads to increase in spead width of 0.5–0.6 mm.
— Diagonal measurements show spread width which is 0.4–0.6 mm bigger than in horizontal and vertical measurements. The bigger the size of the pixel, the greater this variation.
— Measurements near the periphery of the scanning surface show spread width which is 0.4–0.6 mm bigger than measurements near the center.
— Measurements of the X-ray tube at the end of the exploitation period show 0.3–0.6-mm widening of the spread in relation to measurements of the new X-ray tube.

4 Discussion

Image contour spread is taken into account at examination of the spatial resolution, improvement of visualization of small objects, and precision of quantitative CT measurements. Initially, its presence in cranial examinations is discussed [8]. The transition is examined by counting pixels with varying values between the two surrounding constant densities [6, 10]. Such data is used to establish optimal windows and centers for linear measurements [13, 19]. Later the transition layer is represented as a densoprofile [7, 12]. We have also worked out and used our own densoprofile method [17] because of its high precision and easy performance.

Our investigations on spread were aimed at defining its width in practice in connection with optimization of linear measurements of anatomical structures from the CT image [17]. We examined transition layers with sharp edges, i.e., the "ideal" case ensuring minimal spread in relation to the scanned object. The two density ranges (30–80 HU and 800–1200 HU) correspond to density differences

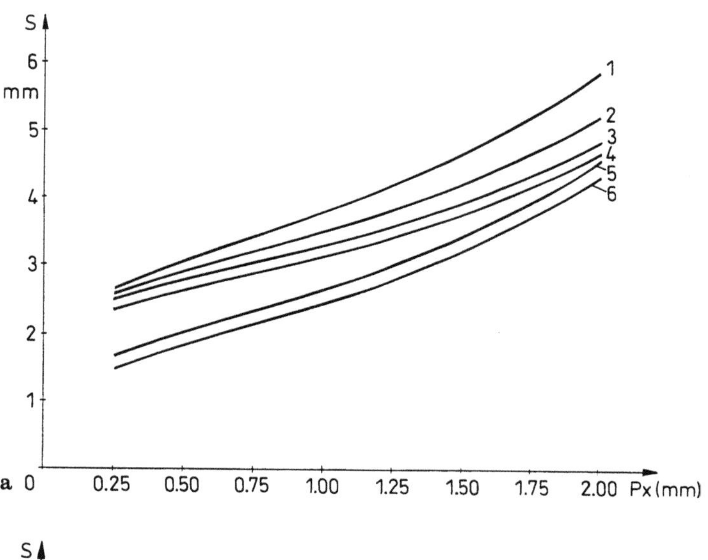

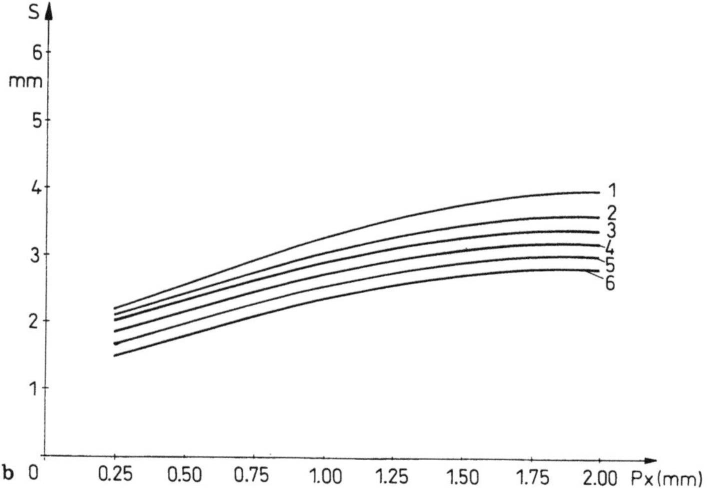

Fig. 2 a, b. Averaged results for image contour spread(S) in computed tomography dependent on pixell(Px) size. **a** 10-mm slice thickness; **b** 5-mm slice thickness. Numbers *1-6* indicates: *1*, density gradient of 800–1200 HU low-frequency (LF) filter; *2*, density gradient of 80–120 HU, LF filter; *3*, density gradient of 800–1200 HU, standard filter; *4*, density gradient of 80–120 HU, standard filter; *5*, density gradient of 800–1200 HU, high-frequency (HF) filter; *6*, density gradient of 80–120 HU, HF filter

most often encountered—soft tissues and fluids, and high density gradient objects in respect to the surrounding medium (bone muscle, trachea/air etc.).

Examination of the transition layer width is the same as examination of impulse response function, but we selected the first term as it is more easily accepted in medical practice. The above-mentioned function is used mainly in defining spatial resolution of the image, specific methods existing for this purpose in CT [2, 5, 12,

20]. Thus it is clear that factors having influence on spread width are the same as these, influencing spatial resolution in CT [15]. In this connection it is evident that spread width increases with increase of pixel size. This increase is approximately linear for pixels of 0.25–1.5 mm, and from 1.5 to 2 mm pixel size depends on slice width. The last fact could be interrelated with decreased quantum density on the X-ray beam for thick slices, beam collimation and detector efficiency, their influence on spatial resolution being known [1]. Due to this, greater spread width (i.e., increased unsharpness) for thick slices can easily be explained. Results for transition layer width for 1.5-mm slices (CE 10 000) are almost the same as those for 5-mm slices, although additional decrease in spread should be expected. This is due to decreased dynamics of the detector signal for this layer with the CE 10000. Spread for the thinnest slices from different CT apparatuses differs considerably because these slices vary from 1 to 3 mm for different X-ray does and detector dynamics, but still we have not measured spread below 0.5 mm for 0.25 mm pixels. It is natural that in the new CT scanner generations this limit will be lower.

Another factor having a strong influence on the transition layer is reconstructive filter type. We measured 1 to 2-mm narrowing of the transition layer when passing from low-frequency to high-frequency reconstructive filter. Usage of special high frequency filters is usually combined with "jumps" (undershots and overshots) at the two ends of a densoprofile showing the transition layer [17, 24]. That is why, in spite of increased slope of the transition layer, we cannot accept the existence of additional spread decrease (because the distance between the two constant densities does not vary essentially). The visual edge-enhancing effect from these filters makes some authors recommend linear measurements for images treated with high-frequency filters [21].

Increase in density gradient (from between 30 and 120 HU to between 800 and 1200 HU) between transition-forming bodies leads to 0.3 to 0.5-mm widening with all other conditions preserved. Nevertheless, results from linear measurements of structures with a great density gradient in relation to the surrounding medium appear to have a great degree of error [4, 18]. The last fact is a consequence of the mutual influence of visualization parameters (window and center) and spread width on visible dimensions of objects [17].

Increase of transition layer width with decrease of the number of projections (decrease in scanning time) and proximity to the periphery of the scanning-surface could be explained with decrease in projection "density" in these cases.

Increased spread in diagonal measurements in comparison with horizontal and vertical measurements is simply explained. The same effect at the end of the exploitation period of the X-ray tube is related, according to us, to increased noise—hence the appearance of jumps at both ends of the densoprofile. The influence of decreased X-ray dose and beam hardness is similar [17].

Secondary processing of CT images—matrix filtration, interpolation, etc.—also leads to increase of spread (to a small extent an exception to this is some special high-frequency matrix filters), but the final effect is strongly dependent on the mathematical apparatus used. The most frequent method for geometric image zooming increases spread width by two to several times. Considerably increased spread in secondary reconstructed (sagital, coronal, etc.) images is not commented on, as they are "rough" in principle and are strongly dependent on the method of acquisition and selection of primary axial slices.

From the various investigations, we established the considerable width and strong variability of the transition layer (from 1.5 to 6 mm on average), dependent on different apparatus parameters. It is natural to raise the question of how such a wide transition layer is visualized—it is expected that on the border of two contiguous bodies a band with gradually varying intensity (optical density) would be observed. In practice when observing such varying gray gradation Mach visual effect appears, thus emphasizing contrast transition (similar to high-frequency filtration), which leads to visual "compression" of the width of this band (the transition layer) [17]. Due to this particular reason it is possible to investigate the transition layer only by densoprofile.

As we said at the beginning, our investigations concern the "ideal" transition layer—i.e., sharp density transition. In practice examined anatomical structures always have rounded contours, which creates in their image contours an extra effect of partial volume. Not dealing here with this effect, already discussed by many authors [9, 16, 22], we shall just point out that it creates an extra increase in spread. Dependent on real object contours, density gradient, slice width, etc., the transition layer width is considerably increased (sometimes more than twice). The effect is even more strongly expressed if the objects "enter at an angle in the slice." This leads to measuring the spread of anatomical object contours from 2 to 12–15 mm (at different apparatus parameters). The above values could be increased due to artifacts and other information distortions.

5 Conclusion

The above-described investigation shows the strong influence of the factors of calculative unsharpness on spread of object contours in CT. The last fact is of particular importance to medical practice—our investigation showed that its neglect of quantitative measurements from the CT image is one of the essential reasons for increased error [17]. The smaller the investigated anatomical object, the greater the error, as spread width becomes comparable and even greater than object size.

Having in mind some general principles of visual information processing we could conclude that such an increased spread exists to a different degree in all modern medical imaging apparatuses with digital image processing. This should be considered in practice, as it could become a source of diagnostic problems, especially in defining dimensions and other parameters of imaged anatomical structures.

6 Summary

Contour spread of visualized objects in computed tomography (CT) is considerably greater than spread in conventional roentgenology. This is due mainly to the specific method for CT, "calculative" unsharpness. Through densoprofile investigation of images of objects with very sharp density transition scanned at different apparatus parameters it is determined that the mean width of contour spread for visualized objects in CT is from 1.5 to 6 mm. Most strongly influencing this spread are the pixel size, the reconstruction filter, the slice width, and the density gradient. Real anatomical object contours are rounded. That additionally widens spread due to the effect of "partial volume" at their edges. Thus, in medical practice this spread varies often from 2 to 12–15 mm, which causes errors during quantitative information extraction from the CT image. That is why spread width should be taken into account especially in diagonistic imaging of small anatomical structures.

References

1. Alexander J, Kalender W, Linke G (1986) Comuptertomographie. Siemens AG, Berlin
2. Assimakopoulos P, Boyd D, Jaschke W, Lipton J (1986) Spatial resolution analysis of computed tomographic images. Invest Radiol 21:260
3. Barett H, Swindell W (1981) Radiological imaging. Academic, New York
4. Beers G, Carter A, Leiter B, Tilak S, Shah R (1985) Interobserver discrepancies in distance measurements from lumbar spine CT scans. AJR 144:395
5. Bentzen S (1983) Evaluation of the spatial resolution of CT scanner by direct analysis of the edge response function. Med Phys 10:579
6. DiChiro G, Arimitsu T, Brooks R (1979) Computed tomography profiles of periventricular hypodensity in hydrocephalus and leukoencephalopathy. Radiology 130:661
7. Eubanks B, Cann C, Zavadski M (1985) CT measurement of the diameter of spinal and other bony canals: effects of section angle and thickness. Radiology 157:243
8. Gado M, Phelps M (1975) The peripheral zone of increased density in cranial computed tomography. Radiology 117:71
9. Goodenough G, Weaver K, Davis D, LaFalse S (1982) Volume averaging limitations of computed tomography. AJR 138:313
10. Jensen P, Orphanoudakis S, Rauschnoeb E, Baron R, Lang R, Rasmussen H (1980) Assessment of bone mass in the radius by computed tomography. AJR 134:285
11. Judy P (1976) The line spread function and modulation transfer function of a computed tomographic scanner. Med Phys 3:233
12. Judy P, Swensson R (1985) Detection of small focal lesions in CT images—Effects of reconstruction filters and visual display windows. Br J Radiol 58:137
13. Koehler P, Anderson R, Baxter B (1979) The effect of computed tomography viewer controls on anatomical measurements. Radiology 130:189
14. Krestel E (1980) Bildgebende Systeme fur die medizinische Diagnostik. Siemens AG, Berlin
15. McCullough E, Payne T, Baker H, Hattery R, Sheedy P, Stephens D, Gedgandus E (1976) Performance evaluation and quality assurance of computed tomography scanners with illustration from the EMI, ACTA and Delta scanners. Radiology 120:173
16. Siegelman S, Zerhouny E, Leo F, Khouri N, Stick F (1980) CT of solitary pulmonary nodule. AJR 135:1
17. Tabakoff S (1988) Optimization of computed tomographic linear and density measurements in medical practice. PhD Dissertation, Sofia
18. Tellkamp H, Rosenkranz G, Geissler S, Hupke M (1987) Die Genauigkeit von computertomographischen Gröpenbestimmungen. Radiol Diagn 28:715
19. Ullrich C, Binet E, Saneski M, Kiefler S (1980) Quantitative assessment of the lumbar spinal canal by computed tomography. Radiology 134:137
20. White D, Speller R, Taylor P (1981) Evaluating performance characteristics in computerized tomography. Br J Radiol 54:221
21. Young S, Nassi M (1985) The critical importance of convolution function (algorithm) selection in the measurment of blood flow in small blood vessels by computed tomography scanning. Comput Radiol 9:287
22. Zhu X (1983) Partial volume phenomenon. AJR 141:842

Frontiers in European Radiology

Editors-in-Chief: A. L. Baert, F. H. W. Heuck

Volume 7

1990. III, 128 pp. 62 figs. 13 tabs.
Hardcover DM 98,– ISBN 3-540-52515-7

A. P. G. van Gils et al.: Non-invasive Imaging of Functioning Paragangli-
omas (Including Phaeochromocytomas). – *W. A. Kaiser:* Dynamic Magnetic Resonance Breast Imaging Using a Double Breast Coil: An Important Step Towards Routine Examination of the Breast. – *H. Bosmans
et al.:* Magnetic Resonance Angiography: Techniques, Prospects, and
Limitations. – *C. Delcour et al.:* Angiographic Evaluation of Impotent
Men. – *G. Wilms et al.:* Laser-Assisted Angioplasty: State of the Art and
Future Developments. – *C. Masciocchi et al.:* The Painful Shoulder:
Magnetic Resonance Imaging Findings.

Volume 6

1989. III, 87 pp. 43 figs. in 100 sep. illus. 15 tabs.
Hardcover DM 118,– ISBN 3-540-50466-4

Magnetic Resonance Imaging of Focal Lesions of Liver and Spleen
Using Gradient-Echo Sequences at 1.5 Tesla:
A Comparison with Ultrasound and Sequential
Computerized Tomography. *J. Griebel,
C. F. Hess, and B. Kurtz.* – Analysis of the Signal
Intensity of FLASH and FISP Fast-Imaging
Pulse Sequences. *S. H. Heywang,
G. Kroebrunner, and M. W. Bauer.* – Ultrasound
of the Hip Joint: Experimental and Clinical
Studies. *R. Langer.* – Defecography: A Supple-
mentary Diagnostic Asset in the Study of the
Disorders of Defecation. *P. H. G. Mahieu.*

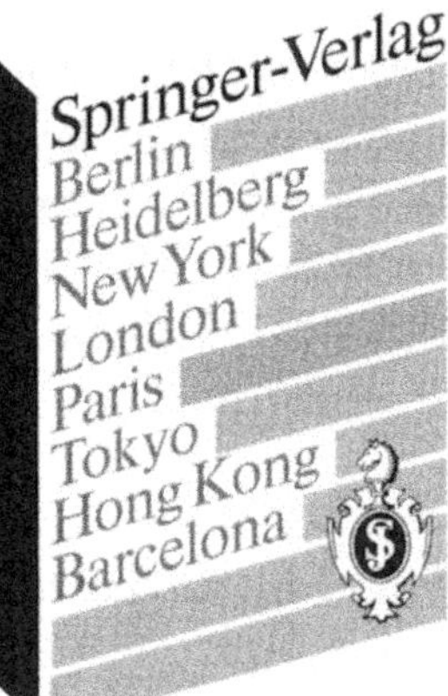

Frontiers in European Radiology

Editors-in-Chief: A. L. Baert, F. H. W. Heuck

Volume 5

1987. III, 176 pp. 120 figs. in 215 sep. illus. 33 tabs.
Hardcover DM 180,- ISBN 3-540-17636-5

Angiocinedensitometry of Renal Blood Circulation by Electrocardio-
gram-Controlled Injection and Computer-Assisted Evaluation. *J. Buck.* –
Experimental Basis of Percutaneous Transluminal Angioplasty.
Ch. L. Zollikofer. – Ultrasound Examination of the Breast – Diagnostic
Information Related to Mammography. *J. Pirschel.* – Computerized
Tomography in Pituitary Microadenoma. *D. Poos and P. Capesius.*

Volume 4

1984. I, 158 pp. 82 figs. in 144 sep. illus.
Hardcover DM 86,- ISBN 3-540-13410-7

Therapeutic Angiography in Neuroradiology: Clinical Objectives and
Results. *P. Lasjaunias, P. Halim, and L. Lopez-Ibor.* – Densitometric
Investigations of Renal Perfusion by Dynamic
X-Ray Computed Tomography. *U. Reiser,
J. Buck, and F. H. W. Heuck.* – Percutaneous
Transhepatic Drainage: Technique, Results,
and Special Applications. *R. Köster.* – Video-
densitometric Measurements of the Blood
Flow in the Model Circulation and in the Iliac
Arteries: Methodological Investigations.
H. Fröhlich.

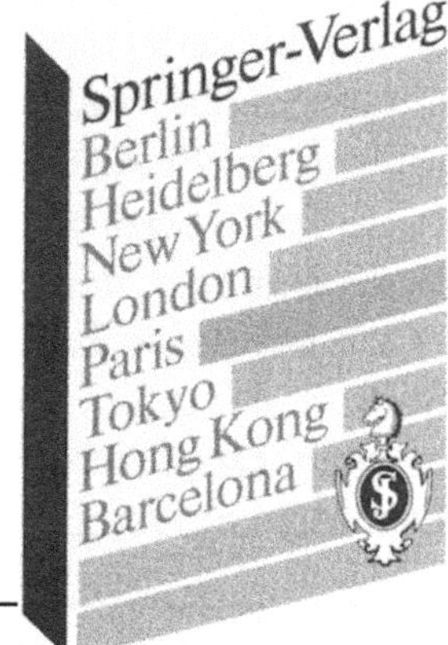

Prices are subject to change without notice.

GPSR Compliance
The European Union's (EU) General Product Safety Regulation (GPSR) is a set
of rules that requires consumer products to be safe and our obligations to
ensure this.

If you have any concerns about our products, you can contact us on

ProductSafety@springernature.com

In case Publisher is established outside the EU, the EU authorized
representative is:

Springer Nature Customer Service Center GmbH
Europaplatz 3
69115 Heidelberg, Germany